UROLOGY
AND PSYCHOSOCIAL ASPECTS
OF CHRONIC, CRITICAL,
AND TERMINAL ILLNESS

UROLOGY AND PSYCHOSOCIAL ASPECTS OF CHRONIC, CRITICAL, AND TERMINAL ILLNESS

Edited by

JOHN K. LATTIMER

PETER DeSANCTIS

MYRON S. ROBERTS

AUSTIN H. KUTSCHER

MAHLON S. HALE

PAUL R. PATTERSON

With the Editorial Assistance of
Lillian G. Kutscher

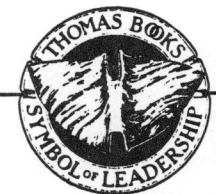

CHARLES C THOMAS • PUBLISHER
Springfield • Illinois • U.S.A.

Published and Distributed Throughout the World by
CHARLES C THOMAS • PUBLISHER
2600 South First Street
Springfield, Illinois, 62717, U.S.A.

This book is protected by copyright. No part of it may be reproduced in any manner without written permission from the publisher.

© *1983 by* CHARLES C THOMAS • PUBLISHER
ISBN 0-398-04729-4
Library of Congress Catalog Card Number: 82-10267

With THOMAS BOOKS *careful attention is given to all details of manufacturing and design. It is the Publisher's desire to present books that are satisfactory as to their physical qualities and artistic possibilities and appropriate for their particular use.* THOMAS BOOKS *will be true to those laws of quality that assure a good name and good will.*

Printed in the United States of America
CU-R-1

Library of Congress Cataloging in Publication Data
Main entry under title:

Urology and psychosocial aspects of chronic, critical, and terminal illness.

Bibliography: p.
Includes index.
1. Genito-urinary organs--Diseases--Psychological aspects. 2. Genito-urinary organs--Diseases--Social aspects. 3. Terminal care. 4. Terminally ill children.
I. Lattimer, John. [DNLM: 1. Urologic diseases.
2. Terminal care--Psychology. 3. Chronic disease--Psychology. 4. Critical care--Psychology. WJ 100 U793]
RC872.U76   1982   616.6   82-10267
ISBN 0-398-04729-4

CONTRIBUTORS

JOHN K. LATTIMER, M.D., Sc.D., Professor and Chairman, Department of Urology, College of Physicians and Surgeons, Columbia University

PETER N. DeSANCTIS, M.D., Assistant Clinical Professor, Department of Urology, College of Physicians and Surgeons, Columbia University

MYRON S. ROBERTS, M.D., Associate Clinical Professor, Department of Urology, College of Physicians and Surgeons, Columbia University

AUSTIN H. KUTSCHER, D.D.S., Professor of Dentistry (in Psychiatry), Department of Psychiatry, College of Physicians and Surgeons, Columbia University; Professor of Dentistry (in Psychiatry), School of Dental and Oral Surgery, Columbia University

MAHLON S. HALE, M.D., Associate Professor, Department of Psychiatry, University of Connecticut Health Science Center

PAUL R. PATTERSON, M.D., Emeritus Professor of Pediatrics, Albany Medical School of Union University

* * * * * * * *

ARTHUR M. ARKIN, M.D., Adjunct Attending Psychiatrist, Montefiore Hospital and Medical Center, Bronx, New York

CHARLTON P. ARMSTRONG, M.D., F.A.C.S., Consulting Senior Associate, Greenville Hospital System; St. Francis Community Hospital; Shriners Hospital for Crippled Children, Greenville, South Carolina

SUCHA O. ASBELL, M.D., Chairperson, Division of Radiation Therapy, Albert Einstein Medical Center, Philadelphia, Pennsylvania; Clinical Assistant Professor, Temple University School of Medicine, Philadelphia, Pennsylvania

LEAH BECK, M.D., Assistant Professor of Clinical Psychiatry, College of Physicians and Surgeons, Columbia University; Consultant, Children's Urology Service, Babies Hospital, Columbia-Presbyterian Medical Center, New York, New York

ESTHER BRAUN, A.C.S.W., Department of Social Service, Babies Hospital, Columbia-Presbyterian Medical Center, New York, New York

ELLIOT L. COHEN, M.D., F.A.C.S., formerly, Chief, Department of Urology, U.S. Public Health Service Hospital, Staten Island, New York; Assistant Professor of Clinical Urology, The Mount Sinai Hospital and Medical School, New York, New York

MARY A. CSENSITS, R.N., E.T., St. Luke's Hospital, Bethlehem, Pennsylvania

BRUCE L. DANTO, M.D., Associate Professor of Psychiatry, Wayne State University School of Medicine, Detroit, Michigan

JACQUELYN EDWARDS, M.S.W., A.C.S.W., University of Texas Cancer Center, M.D. Anderson Hospital and Tumor Institute, Houston, Texas

WILLIAM F. FINN, M.D., Attending Gynecologist, North Shore University Hospital, Manhasset, New York; Associate Professor of Obstetrics and Gynecology, Cornell University Medical College, New York, New York

JAMES F. GLENN, M.D., F.A.C.S., Professor of Surgery (Urology) and Dean, School of Medicine, Emory University, Atlanta, Georgia

TERRY W. HENSLE, M.D., Assistant Professor of Clinical Urology, College of Physicians and Surgeons, Columbia University, New York, New York

JOHN D. JEFFERIES, M.D., Assistant Professor of Surgery and Neurology, University of Connecticut Health Science Center, Farmington, Connecticut

KATHERINE F. JETER, Ed.D., E.T., Assistant Clinical Professor of Urology, Medical University of South Carolina, Charleston, South Carolina

GEORGE KRUPP, M.D., D.M.Sc., Psychiatric Consultant, Bereavement Center of Family Service Association, Hempstead, New York

HARLAN A. KUTSCHER, M.D., Attending Urologist, Saint Joseph Hospital, Reading, Pennsylvania

LILLIAN G. KUTSCHER, Publications Editor, The Foundation of Thanatology, New York, New York

CAROL LANDAU, A.C.S.W., Coordinator, Geriatrics Mental Health Clinic, South Nassau Communities Hospital, Oceanside,

New York
SUSAN P. LEVINE, M.D., Assistant Professor of Psychiatry, University of Illinois Medical School, Chicago, Illinois
ARNOLD MELMAN, M.D., Department of Urology, Beth Israel Hospital and Medical Center, New York, New York
RABBI STEVEN A. MOSS, Coordinator, Jewish Chaplaincy Services, Memorial Sloan-Kettering Cancer Center, New York, New York; Spiritual Leader, B'nai Israel Reform Temple, Oakdale, New York
HYMAN L. MUSLIN, M.D., Professor of Psychiatry, University of Illinois Medical School, Chicago, Illinois
EDWIN NADEL, Chartered Life Underwriter, New York, New York
JOHN J. PARKER, Esq., Attorney at Law, New York, New York
DIANNE BARTH PIERSON, M.D., Psychiatry Service, Veterans Administration Medical Center, Gainesville, Florida
LINDA M. RHODES, Ed.D., Consultant, Center for Geriatrics and Gerontology, Faculty of Medicine, Columbia University, New York, New York
GERALD ROSNER, A.M., Chartered Life Underwriter, Executive Director, P.M. Planning Co., New York, New York; Adjunct Associate Professor, The College of Insurance, New York, New York
GEORGE SAENZ, M.S.W., A.C.S.W., University of Texas Cancer Center, M.D. Anderson Hospital and Tumor Institute; Veterans Administration Medical Center, Houston, Texas
CHARLES D. SAUNDERS, M.D., F.A.C.S., Clinical Associate Professor of Urology, Temple University School of Medicine, Philadelphia, Pennsylvania; Chief, Division of Urology, St. Luke's Hospital, Bethlehem, Pennsylvania
MORRIS J. SCHOENEMAN, M.D., Assistant Professor of Pediatric Nephrology, Mount Sinai School of Medicine, New York, New York
JEROME J. SPUNBERG, M.D., Attending Staff Physician, Division of Radiation Therapy, Albert Einstein Medical Center, Philadelphia, Pennsylvania; Clinical Assistant Professor, Temple University School of Medicine, Philadelphia, Pennsylvania
REGE SZUTS STEWART, M.D., Department of Psychiatry, Southwestern Medical School, University of Texas Health Science Center, Dallas, Texas

KATHLEEN A. WEBER, R.N., M.P.H., formerly, Coordinator, Cancer Support Program, U.S. Public Health Service Hospital, Staten Island, New York

HANS H. ZINSSER, M.D., Professor of Urology, College of Physicians and Surgeons, Columbia University (deceased)

PREFACE

IN caring for the patient with primary urological pathology or complications resulting from disease in other organ systems, the urologists' goals are to combine in equal measures the art and the science of their professional skill. Without the surgical techniques derived from scientific training, they can offer no hope of relief or cure to the patient. However, without a substantial measure of empathic care, they can compromise the patient's acceptance of the quality of life being supported. When the body's mechanical dysfunction can be repaired or restored only partially, the patient may have real difficulty in adjusting to life as it must thereafter be lived. Supportive care then becomes a challenge to the urologist, the staff, and the patient's family.

At whatever age a patient is deprived of any aspect of normal urologic function, the results can be particularly devastating. Incontinence, sexual dysfunction, pain, and organ failure all impose suffering that extends beyond physical dimensions to alter interpersonal connections of the most intimate nature. As those who have contributed to this book demonstrate, the somatic and psychic impact of urological pathology compounds the indignities that illness imposes.

It is the purpose of this book to focus on the psychosocial aspects of the care to be offered this special group of patients and their family members by the supporting team, which includes the urologist, the psychiatrist, the psychologist, the nurse, the ostomy specialist, and the social worker, as well as by the clergyperson and other counselors from medical and nonmedical disciplines. No matter how guarded the prognosis in terms of normal function or life span, there is little doubt that the sensitive professional can provide an extra dimension of care in ways that can ease the suffering of the body, the mind, and the spirit.

John K. Lattimer

ACKNOWLEDGMENT

THE focus of the discipline of thanatology is on the art of enhancing humanitarian caregiving for patients who are critically, chronically, or terminally ill, with equal concern exhibited for the well-being of their family members. From a base in thanatology, interdisciplinary professionals are dedicated to promoting vastly improved psychosocial and medical care for these patients and assistance for their families. Proposed is a philosophy of caregiving that reinforces alternative ways of supporting positive qualities in the dying patient's life and that introduces methods of intervention on behalf of the emotional support of his or her family members and bereaved survivors.

The editors wish to acknowledge the support and encouragement of The Foundation of Thanatology in the preparation of this volume. All royalties from the sale of this book are assigned to The Foundation of Thantology, a tax exempt, not for profit, public, scientific, and educational foundation.

CONTENTS

	Page
Preface	v

John K. Lattimer

I.
AN OVERVIEW OF PATIENT CARE

Chapter

1. HELPING THE PATIENT TO LIVE WITH DIGNITY AND MEANING DURING THE LIVING-DYING PHASE OF HIS ILLNESS.............. 5
   Charlton P. Armstrong
2. THE PHYSICIAN AS SCIENTIST AND HEALER.................... 15
   Dianne Barth Pierson
3. THE CLERGYMAN AND THE CARE OF THE POSTOPERATIVE PATIENT 20
   Steven A. Moss
4. CARING — THE HEART OF OSTOMY NURSING.................. 25
   Mary A. Csensits
5. TREATMENT OF THE CANCER PATIENT BY THE PRIMARY CARE PHYSICIAN... 35
   Hyman L. Muslin and Susan P. Levine
6. THE ROLE OF GROUP PROCESS IN STAFF SURVIVAL WITH THE DYING PATIENT.. 49
   Mahlon S. Hale and John D. Jefferies
7. THE FUNCTIONING OF AN ETHICS COMMITTEE IN A COMMUNITY HOSPITAL... 58
   William F. Finn

II.
SPECIFIC PROBLEMS IN UROLOGIC CAREGIVING

8. SELF-IDENTIFIED FEARS AND CONCERNS OF BLADDER CANCER

Chapter	Page
PATIENTS	65
George Saenz and Jacquelyn Edwards	
9. CARE OF DYING PATIENTS WITH INCIDENTAL BLADDER OUTLET OBSTRUCTION	72
Harlan A. Kutscher	
10. BENEMORTASIA	75
Charles D. Saunders	
11. UROLOGICAL CARE OF THE TERMINAL CANCER PATIENT	80
Elliot L. Cohen	
12. A HOSPITAL CANCER SUPPORT GROUP	83
Kathleen A. Weber	
13. URINARY INCONTINENCE	86
Katherine F. Jeter	
14. URINARY TRACT DISABILITY	90
Peter N. DeSanctis	
15. PSYCHOSOCIAL ASPECTS OF THE RADIOTHERAPEUTIC MANAGEMENT OF UROGENITAL MALIGNANCY	97
Jerome J. Spunberg and Sucha O. Asbell	
16. DIABETES, IMPOTENCE, AND SEXUALITY	104
Arnold Melman	
17. MECHANICAL ASPECTS OF RESTORATION OF SEXUAL FUNCTION IN THE DISABLED MALE PATIENT	109
James F. Glenn	
18. THE DEPARTING GERIATRIC PATIENT	113
Hans H. Zinsser	
19. ANTICIPATORY GRIEVING AND COGNITIVE MASTERY IN THE MANAGEMENT OF THE PSYCHOLOGICAL ASPECTS OF KIDNEY REJECTION	117
Rege Szuts-Stewart	
20. PSYCHOLOGICAL ASPECTS OF CHRONIC HEMODIALYSIS AND PSYCHIATRIC COMPLICATIONS OF THE PATIENT: A REVIEW OF THE LITERATURE	123
Linda M. Rhodes	

III.
THE PEDIATRIC UROLOGY PATIENT

Chapter

21. EMOTIONAL EFFECTS OF CHRONIC UROLOGIC ILLNESS ON
    CHILDREN 153
    Leah Beck
22. THE ROLE OF SOCIAL WORK IN THE CARE OF THE SERIOUSLY
    ILL CHILD UROLOGY PATIENT 158
    Esther Braun
23. THE CHILD WITH UROLOGIC CANCER 170
    Terry W. Hensle
24. CHILDREN WITH UROLOGIC PROBLEMS: PSYCHOLOGICAL
    NEEDS 174
    Katherine F. Jeter
25. PSYCHOSOCIAL PROBLEMS OF THE CHILD AND FAMILY
    UNDERGOING DIALYSIS AND TRANSPLANTATION 179
    Morris J. Schoeneman

IV.
PSYCHOSOCIAL CONSIDERATIONS FOR THE PATIENT AND THE FAMILY

26. THE PATIENT'S FREEDOM IN DECISION MAKING 189
    Bruce L. Danto
27. ESTATE PLANNING FOR THE TERMINALLY ILL 196
    Gerald Rosner
28. EMOTIONAL CARE OF THE BEREAVED 201
    Arthur M. Arkin
29. VARIANTS OF PATHOLOGICAL BEREAVEMENT 207
    George Krupp and Carol Landau
30. A CONFIDENTIAL FAMILY CHECKLIST 223
    Edwin Nadel and John J. Parker

Index 233

UROLOGY
AND PSYCHOSOCIAL ASPECTS
OF CHRONIC, CRITICAL,
AND TERMINAL ILLNESS

I.
AN OVERVIEW OF PATIENT CARE

Chapter 1

HELPING THE PATIENT TO LIVE WITH DIGNITY AND MEANING DURING THE LIVING–DYING PHASE OF HIS ILLNESS

CHARLTON P. ARMSTRONG

DEATH and dying are not synonymous, but distinct and separate events. About death we know little; even the clinical definition of it is ambiguous. Moreover, about death, almost nothing can be known apart from religious faith or parapsychology. About dying, a great deal can be learned and shared, since a pattern for dying is formed and exhibited in the behavior of persons engaged in the process. "Death itself is not a problem of life, for death is not amenable to treatment or intervention. We may consider death only as an issue between man and God. But the process of dying is very much a part of a person's life" (Pattison, 1977, p. 43).

This is not to suggest that death as a metaphysical problem is of no interest to physicians. We are mortal, too, and the realization of our own mortality is as likely to introduce the metaphysical question to our minds as it is to the mind of the layman. Despite protests and reassurances to the contrary, it is likely that the most disturbing fact about our existence is contemplation of the possibility of our nonexistence.

However, this is not a paper on the nature of death, but about what Mansell Pattison has called "the living–dying interval" (p. 44). All living persons are dying, to be sure, but only those confronted by crisis knowledge of death's reality may be expected to need the physician's special care in coping with the living–dying phase of their illness. Disease originating in or involving the genitourinary tract is the particular focus of this presentation. We are considering the main malignancy and its consequences. The thesis argued here is that the physician's role with such patients is not only the exercise of his professional skill to conquer the disease or to care for the patient during the final resolution of the disease if it remains unconquered, but to provide support and guidance in the living–dying interval, however long or short that may be, so that the quality of the patient's life may be as rich as possible during the process.

Certain distressing physiological accompaniments to the presence and treatment of carcinoma of the genitourinary tract, so-called *side effects* causing acute distress to the patient and diverting his attention from the primary struggle, will be briefly commented upon. Among such side effects are the following: (1) unexpected complications from radiation therapy; (2) loss or diminution of the sexual function, creating anxiety and depression, especially as related to the patient's spouse; and (3) social embarrassment from the effects of urinary incontinence with resulting odor, etc. Next, attention will be called to certain emotional and psychic needs of the patient who knows that he is suffering a life-threatening disease and is passing through the living–dying interval. Included are (1) anxiety about the unknown and the uncertain, (2) the temptation to lapse into regression and helplessness, (3) depression and the importance of the maintenance of hope, and (4) the need of the physician to enlist the continuing assistance and support of significant others in the care of the patient. Finally, I shall comment upon the signal importance of the physician–patient relationship during the living–dying phase of the patient's illness.

Side Effects Causing Distress and Diverting Attention

Postponement of death may be achieved at a cost so great to the patient's quality of life that the treatment itself should be under review. Presumably, most patients would elect life at any price, but the distress caused by some treatment tends to divert the patient and the doctor from the main struggle, control or eradication of the disease.

Among the side effects that we see in our work with patients who have been treated with external beam radiation for carcinoma of the genitourinary tract and, in particular, of the prostate is obstruction of lymphatic channels, resulting in localized fluid retention and marked edema that generally are irreversible. Of course, the most common site for spontaneous blockage by tumor is the lower extremity. I am speaking particularly about edema of the penis and scrotum, which may become quite massive. Prolonged postoperative drainage after lymph node dissection offers the active patient both diversion and distress.

Another complication of radiation is the subsequent development of a "cord" bladder, even diverting the attention of a patient from a Stage C undifferentiated carcinoma of the prostate. As we all are aware, the most common complications of radiation are those of nausea, vomiting, and diarrhea, and the development of bed sores. The latter complication, of course, seems to appear often in overweight patients and sometimes necessitates plastic surgical repair. An extremely depressing complication capable of diverting attention would include the appearance of vesicovaginal and vesicolic fistulae and sequelae. This would compare with a bowel fistula following cystectomy in combination with preoperative and postoperative external beam radiation.

A most startling example of diverting attention from the primary was seen in the elderly patient who, after a radical nephrectomy, developed a tumor embolus to the contralateral kidney with subsequent dialysis over a period of months. There was also a young, successful, physically active executive who developed a metastatic melanoma of the upper urinary tract. Over a period of almost two years, even while the patient pursued nearly normal activities, the patient–family–physician team lived the experience of the tumor constantly moving down stream. Initially, this necessitated surgery on the upper urinary tract, then on the urinary bladder in multiple fashion, and eventually in the distal urethra.

A second side effect of carcinoma of the prostate is the loss of sexual function following radical prostatectomy. Males who have been sexually active often report a severe sense of loss and uneasiness about being unable to have intercourse following this procedure. The primary manifestation of this loss is the sense of deprivation and the anger and resentment accompanying it. To the male whose ability to perform sexually has been an important source of self-esteem as a man, the loss is especially difficult to accept. Careful follow-up indicates a surprisingly high percentage of residual sexual function following radical retropubic prostatectomy. In recent years, the penile prosthesis has been utilized with reasonably good results in carefully selected cases where the patient desires insertion of the prosthesis. The patient's spouse is, in this instance, as in the entire issue of the male patient suffering with the debilitating effects of carcinoma and its treatment, a key person. Her support in the husband's embarrassment and sense of loss of his ability to have satisfactory sexual relations is imperative to a healthy resolution of this aspect of his treatment.

A third side effect of treatment of malignancy of the urinary tract is social embarrassment from incontinence with resultant wetting of clothing, the fear of unpleasant odors, and so forth. Such problems become nagging and persistent annoyances to the patient, causing him to feel insecure in public and diverting his attention from the struggle with his disease. It may be argued that such distractions serve the good purpose of preventing the patient's preoccupation with his degenerating physical condition, but patients suffering from these unpleasant accompaniments of treatment often see them as constant reminders of their condition. Thus, in such patients the physician encounters a high level of frustration and anger because the problem persists.

Emotional Needs of the Patient in the Dying Trajectory

Probably more significant than the physiological side effects of treatment of carcinoma of the genitourinary tract are certain common emotional needs of the patient who senses that he is in a living-dying trajectory. His physician may be of enormous support to him through sensitivity to the presence of these needs, although they may never be spoken of directly by the patient.

Among these emotional crises is anxiety. Any number of physiological factors may introduce to the patient's mind the anxiety that he is gravely ill. Changes in his appearance, feelings of debilitation, loss of weight, pain, and disability may suggest to the patient that things are not well with him. For example, patients whose lives are maintained on hemodialysis live in a world of continuing uncertainty. There is hope for life and fear for death. Their wish is for a return to the state of health they once knew and yet they seem to live with constant sickness. They strive to regain quality but are forced to accept a life of compromised quality. They sense that they live on borrowed time and dying is truly a constant reality. During the chronic phase, the patient faces several anxieties that the physician must be aware of in order to help the patient identify and resolve each specific issue in an appropriate manner.

Among the most frequent of these fears is anxiety about the *unknown*. Diggory and Rothman (Pattison, 1977, p. 49) separate fears of the unknown into the following categories:

1. What life experiences will I not be able to have?
2. What is my fate in the hereafter?
3. What will happen to my body after death?
4. What will happen to my survivors?
5. How will my family and friends respond to my dying?
6. What will happen to my life plans and projects?
7. What changes will occur in my body?
8. What will be my emotional reactions?

It is plain that some of the above anxieties about the unknown can be answered by the physician, and some cannot. Moreover, some are unanswerable. Although the physician is aware of such questions in the patient's mind and does not raise them himself, by being ready to accept them and deal with them appropriately when the patient raises them, he is able to be of enormous help to the patient in this phase of his trajectory.

Other fears include *loneliness*. There is a feeling of isolation from oneself and others which accompanies long-term illness. This is aided and abetted by the avoidance behavior of others in their dealing with the gravely ill person. They do not want to bother him, which is a way of rationalizing behavior that reflects their own discomfort in the presence of such gravity. The sense of isolation is not only psychological, but in our culture (which turns over to the medical facilities the responsibility for care of the dying) it may also be physical. Much of the problem of the hospital's isolation of the dying patient revolves around the purpose of the hospital, which is curative in function rather than caring. The dying person needs a great deal of care when cure is no longer an option of the hospitalization.

Necessary withdrawal from work or recreational activities, long before the patient becomes hospitalized, may begin the process of isolation and loneliness. The living–dying patient senses that he is slowly but surely being cut off from the everyday associations that gave him a sense of identity and place. If his physician listens for his patient's signals, he may well hear loneliness as part of the heaviness borne by the patient in his life trajectory toward death.

Other fears include the *anticipatory grief* of the patient who begins to experience the sense of impending loss of family and friends ahead of time—his own death cutting him off from all that he holds dear. In the poignant chronicle of his losing battle against leukemia, which he entitled *Stay of Execution*, the late Stewart Alsop recorded his feelings of loss movingly: "And then a sense of the reality of death crowded in on me—the end of a pleasant life, never to see Tish or Andrew or Nicky or the four older children again, never to go to Needwood again, or laugh with friends, or see the spring come. There came upon me a terrible sense of aloneness, of vulnerability, of nakedness, of helplessness" (1973, p. 68).

Other fears we commonly are in touch with as we care for the living-dying patient are fear of loss of self-determination, fear of the pain and suffering that may accompany the progress of his illness, and fear of the changes that are or will be taking place in his body. To be sensitive to such fears in his patient and to be ready to accept the expression of them by the patient is important to the physician's care.

The tendency to regress into a helpless state is a common manifestation of patients in the living-dying trajectory. Regression may have positive as well as negative effects. Among the positive factors is the patient's willingness to accept help from others without undue questioning, and especially to rely upon the authority figure of his physician as the source of wisdom and power. Another aspect of regression in the severely ill patient who has concluded that he is going to die is the tendency to anticipate the future in terms of ever shorter projections. Like the child who can think no further ahead than next week or his birthday, or until next Christmas, so the dying patient shifts his focus from the distant to the immediate future. He counts time in weeks, not years, and learns to cherish and cling to each experience as though it might be his last. The living-dying patient frequently expresses gratitude for the qualitative intensification of his awareness of time and event. It is one of the bonuses of his shortened life expectancy.

The negative aspect of regression has to do with giving up. Occasionally we see the patient who has withdrawn from the commonplace engagements of life—work, play, social engagements—and has accepted a helplessness and hopelessness, which reflect that he or she is no longer willing to make a fight of it. This is the patient who sits alone in a semidarkened room, who sleeps excessively, or who may sit and stare hour after unbroken hour at his television screen. He is no longer trying to hold on to concrete reality or making himself participate in life. This may occur long before physical necessity requires such regression. It is a form of emotional death in anticipation of the physical death of the patient. The regressed patient may resent any intrusion into his little world of certainty. In this sense, regression may be as much a symptom of the illness as the diseased organ, and the physician who realizes what is happening is better prepared to deal with it. For example, the tendency of the regressed patient to reduce the time scale of his expectations may be used by the physician to restore hope. "When you get out of the hospital, I hope you will take that trip you have been talking about." By living on a day-by-day basis, there is the lively potential for a considerable degree of fulfillment and satisfaction of ego needs. As Pattison aptly puts it, "the will to live seems to be associated with having something or someone to live for" (1977, p. 71).

Little is as important in the doctor-patient relationship as the maintenance of hope. Kübler-Ross's work (1969), while subject to considerable question because of its neat categorization of the process of dying into five definitive stages (denial, anger, bargaining, depression, and acceptance), is nonetheless provocative and helpful. There are many cases where the Kübler-Ross stages are not followed; a patient cannot be forced into a particular stage. The patterns cannot be artificial for the individual patient, and the stages are not necessarily chronological. The medical team must respond to where the patient is. From interviews with hundreds of dying patients, Kübler-Ross speaks out strongly about the importance of the maintenance of hope by those who care for the dying. Hope should never be withdrawn from the patient. To tell the patient of the seriousness of his illness is appropriate. To encourage him to hope, to believe in the possibility of further treatment, that all of his options have not been exhausted, and that new discoveries for the treatment of what he has are being made continually are most important for the continued struggle of the patient, and his desire to fight off the depression that threatens to rob him of his will to resist.

In this continuing struggle against what is likely to be an irresistible enemy, significant others such as spouse, children, pastor, priest or rabbi, and close friends are an invaluable ally of the physician. He needs, therefore, to enlist their help in ministering to the patient. Insufficient attention has been given to the dying process as a social interaction. We have focused upon the dying person, but he does not die alone. He dies in relationship with others. To observe only the dying person is to ignore the effect of the dying process upon others involved with the patient, and thus to ignore the impact that these significant others have upon the successful coping of the patient in his living-dying trajectory. The patient's family and significant circle of others need to be involved with the physician in the patient's care.

Physician-Patient Relationship During the Living-Dying Phase

The patient reacts in various ways to his physician's behavior and is, as his disease progresses, increasingly sensitive to the vibrations he picks up or thinks he senses in the physician's manner toward him. Almost any act or statement of the physician may acquire significance far out of proportion to the physician's intention. The patient may be compared to one who is in a state of lonely vigil and growing dependency, sharply observing his doctor, gathering information, and reaching conclusions based upon what he thinks he hears and sees. Even silence may be a meaningful covert communication, saying more than the doctor intends. "Why doesn't he talk to me about what is going on?" may be the patient's evaluation of the relationship between him and his doctor, and he may well jump to the conclusion that nothing is being said to him because the news is all bad. The doctor may never utter the word *incurable*, and yet his manner or failure to reach out to the patient communicates the hopelessness of the situation.

Does the patient want to be told the gravity of his condition? Kübler-Ross is certain that most do; so are Kelly and Friesen (Weir, 1977, pp. 5-6, 15). Doctors who treat cancer patients tend to disagree with those conclusions. Most who have reported their own practice in such matters say that they tell only by bits and pieces, carefully protecting the patient from too severe a burden to his hope for recovery. Joseph Fletcher, a theologian and ethicist, argues that the patient has the right to know "the truth, nothing but the truth, and all the truth" (Weir, p. 28f).

Bernard C. Meyer (Weir, p. 42f) properly says that the question of what to tell the patient about his illness is but one facet of the practice of medicine as an art, a particular example of that spoken and mute dialogue between patient and physician that has always been and will always be an indispensable ingredient in the therapeutic process. "How to carry on this dialogue, what to say and when to say it, and what not to say, are questions not unlike those posed by an awkward suitor." *There are some actions we as physicians must avoid.* We should constantly be aware of and try to avoid stimulation of anxiety in the patient by any statement made without thought. We should avoid any therapeutic ambition that might lead to unnecessary procedures. We must strive for no loss of identity on the part of the patient by encouraging continuing personal contact by family, friends, and ourselves. We must relate to the dying person as a living person. Laurens P. White argues that the doctor may be forthright with his patient without destroying the patient's hope because there is a built-in capacity for hopefulness in most human beings. White quotes one patient friend who "gave me a phrase, an understanding, and a gift which have been central in my life for 25 years. . . . He was dying of melanoma, early in middle life, riddled with metastases which were apparent to him, and not responding to the ineffective drugs then available." This patient said to his physician one day, "You know, Laurie, I know I'm dying, but I don't really believe I'm dying." "In these simple words," White writes, "he gave me an answer to the enigma of denial, and in truth, a solution for dealing with it. . . . I can deal with the patient, being as truthful as I know how to be, and the denial which is built into the patient will enable him or her to deal with the truth" (Feifel, 1977, p. 100).

My own personal conclusion and the intent by which I conduct my practice is to care for my patients, attempting to provide both expert technical care and the involved, concerned human care that every human being desires and deserves. This means helping patients to live as long as they can live and helping them to do so with meaning and dignity. It is also my creed to help people through the living–dying trajectory so that death can be accepted when it becomes inevitable.

References

Alsop, S.: *Stay of Execution.* Philadelphia, J.B. Lippincott Co., 1973, p. 68.
Feifel, H.: *New Meanings of Death.* New York, McGraw-Hill, Inc., 1977, p. 100.

Kübler-Ross, E.: *On Death and Dying*. New York, Macmillan Co., 1969.
Pattison, E.M.: *The Experience of Dying*. Englewood Cliffs, New Jersey, Prentice-Hall, Inc., 1977.
Weir, R.F. (Ed.): *Ethical Issues in Death and Dying*. New York, Columbia University Press, 1977.

Chapter 2

THE PHYSICIAN AS SCIENTIST AND HEALER

DIANNE BARTH PIERSON

THE skepticism of science has eroded the attitude of the physician as healer. The advance of modern technology has caught medicine between attitudes of science and healing. Every physician who becomes involved in the treatment of the terminally ill experiences this dilemma.

The attitude of the physician toward death reflects his attitude toward life. The physician functioning as scientist must from necessity base his outlook on doubt. Empirical knowledge is obtained through skepticism. When doubt looks at death, it sees an unknown force, a dark evil to be avoided at all costs. Doubt generates anxiety; death becomes a feared concept, a tragedy. With an attitude of doubt, the time one lives has priority over the life–death experience. The physician scientist rushes in to "save" the patient from death when terminal illness is discovered, using the defense mechanisms of denial and avoidance. The scientist encourages the acceptance of the death process only when the treatment fails, as a final afterthought, and may experience the death of the patient as his own personal failure. The attitude of doubt sees the physician and the patient as helpless victims of a dreaded disease.

The physician as healer, on the other hand, bases his outlook on the wholeness of life, on an intuitive trust in the totality of existence. Life in its totality does not exist as life alone, but as the life–death experience. Death from the perspective of trust is a natural outcome of life. Rather than a feared tragedy, death is seen as the final challenge to a conscious being. The healer begins treatment with the acceptance of the death process. The initial focus on this challenge to the psyche for growth alleviates psychic feelings of helplessness. The orientation of treatment becomes the quality of the life–death experience rather than the five year survival rate following diagnosis of the disease.

While it is the scientist who uses appropriate medical knowledge to develop treatment modalities for palliative care, it is the healer who aids the patient and the family in the acceptance of the life-death process. A physician needs to be aware of the different attitudes required in each aspect of treatment. The skepticism of science has eroded the attitude of the physician as healer. Neglecting the art of healing is ethically unsound. It creates emotional chaos and disasters of poor communication that add to the burden of suffering of the terminally ill and their families and that cause tension and stress between the patient and the physician during the treatment period.

The art of healing is available to any physician well grounded in an attitude of trust and a consciousness of the totality of existence. The attitude of trust creates a therapeutic situation in which a feeling of personal power is restored to the patient. The decision of how to die gives the concept of death a certain dignity which frees the psyche of overwhelming impotence. The compassion generated between physician and patient through the attitude of trust provides a basis for clear communication during the treatment period.

Approaching the Dying Patient and the Family

The ideal time to begin family therapy is when the diagnosis of terminal illness is made and communicated to the patient. The usual defense mechanisms in dying patients — denial, isolation, avoidance, and withdrawal — are exaggerated when the ordeal of the shock wave is experienced in the context of early onset of medical treatment, when the patient is often alone and away from family members. It is essential to include all family members in treatment. If blood relatives are not available, encourage the patient to include any support group that he considers family, who are willing to function in this capacity during the treatment period. Optimum group size for the initial family session is four to six members, including the patient.

The issue of loss of a member is a great stress upon the family system. Early in the first session, affect distortion and cognitive dissonance may be high. The idea of death triggers psychic processes in every group member. The role of the healer is to facilitate confrontation of the initial issues of death and acceptance. Family members are helpful in clarifying issues for one another. Information given the patient regarding the illness may be discussed and fed back by other family members after meeting with the physician.

The healer, from the perspective of trust, defines grief and introduces the concept of totality into the family system. From the healing perspective, grief is not simply the result of the loss of a loved one, but rather the result of the missed opportunity to love. Families are encouraged to open themselves to an attitude of acceptance of the here and now and to work toward loving each other totally in the time that remains.

The initial family meeting is an act of prevention. Anticipatory grief binds emotional energy in the family system which may present later on as symptoms of psychopathology. Norman Paul and others have discussed various ways in which unresolved grief may manifest, such as addiction, psychosis, depression, neurosis, and physical illness. A wide variety of symptoms may be intricately tied to the issue of loss. When grief is approached through the concept of totality, the family system begins to assume responsibility for the quality of their life-death experience. As the intimacy level rises, the family develops the power to heal itself through the process of acceptance.

After establishing the support system, the physician schedules a second family session to discuss treatment options. Separation of the issues of death and acceptance from those of treatment allows for clarity. The presentation of too much material in the first session will cause the systems to overload. A two- or three-day lag period gives the patient and the family time to process and discuss their feelings and to emerge from the shock wave of discovery before making a rational decision about treatment. The healer, having developed an attitude of trust, will find his role as scientist facilitated. A major factor in the emotional distress of the terminally ill is eliminated when the patient no longer feels locked into a system of isolation and disengagement from family members.

During the second session, the physician presents the facts and figures of treatment and prognosis and the treatment options available. The option of no treatment needs discussion. The psyche needs to know it has a choice in order not to feel overpowered by the forces of death. The right to refuse treatment or to stop treatment at any point allows the patient a sense of mastery over his fate. It is essential to do this initial groundwork to prepare the patient for the eventual side effects that occur with the palliative therapies. For example, at the time of a recurrence of a cancer, the psyche, having the awareness of choice, is free to decide the moment of death with dignity.

The physician may work individually with the patient during the first phase of time-limited chemotherapy or radiotherapy. A third family session is helpful after the first phase of treatment. The family has the opportunity to ask questions, share experiences, and raise any issues that need further discussion. The attitude of trust is the essential key to the family's acceptance of whatever lies ahead. Some families will need no further therapy; others may wish to continue sessions. The physician explores the option of supportive therapy. If indicated, the physician refers the family to any health care professional, chaplain, or significant other of their choice. It is important that the family have some forum to discuss their ideas and feelings about death, particularly when death is imminent. Simply making the patient and the family aware of the need is sometimes adequate. Many family systems are capable of carrying along on their own, once the attitude of trust has been established. For those families who need further therapy, the physician recommends follow-up sessions after the first phase of treatment, at the time of recurrence of the disease, and during the death event. In these families, the training of a therapist may be necessary for maintaining the intimacy level required for the process of acceptance of the death event.

The attitude of doubt as well as that of trust will fluctuate as the family struggles with the issue of grief. The obvious advantage of a family systems approach is that the experience of one family member becomes a model for the others. The affect expressed by one group member triggers an emotional response in another. The intensity of the group experience hammers away at the denial present in the system until, ultimately, all family members begin to express their feelings. When these phenomena occur, the process of acceptance begins. At this point the therapist introduces the concept of totality into the system and defines grief from the healing perspective. The power of healing is restored to the family system when the feeling task is oriented toward the quality of their life–death experience. The immediate rewards in terms of intimacy are self-evident as the family awareness focuses on the opportunity to love. The energy ordinarily bound in anticipatory grief becomes available for the expression of tenderness, love, and affection.

In summary, medical treatment in dying persons requires a fusion of the attitudes of science and healing. In order to be effective, a physician must operate in both spheres. It is time that the attitudes of science and healing work together in order to provide optimum treatment for the terminally ill and their families.

Chapter 3

THE CLERGYMAN AND THE CARE OF THE POSTOPERATIVE PATIENT

STEVEN A. MOSS

AS a professional chaplain, I am often asked by my colleagues who are primarily involved in congregational life and not in hospitals, "What do you do when you visit a person who is hospitalized?" The inadequacy felt by many clergymen regarding their ministrations to the sick is increased when they are confronted by persons who are dying or who are facing catastrophic illness. These anxieties are heightened when the patient's illness brings about visible changes in body image, or demonstrative changes in self-image. It is these changes that ask the visiting clergyman for a response, which is difficult to give.

Why is there difficulty in giving this emotional response to the patient whose body image and self-image have changed? The difficulty might be attributed to the emotional makeup of the clergyman. It might be that as he identifies with the patient, he sees too much of the patient in himself. As he then finds it difficult to establish an empathetic distance, his emotional response becomes more negative than positive. The difficulty in responding to this type of patient might also involve the clergyman's training. After all, how many seminaries have chaplaincy internship programs in their curricula? And how many seminarians prepare their students for the highly specialized ministry needed in caring for the person suffering from catastrophic illness, for the person who is dying?

Confronting the question of the proper way for seminaries to prepare clergymen for their professional life is one way of dealing with this ministerial problem. But what about the clergyman out of seminary? What can be done for him? I would suggest that he obtain experience by participating in a chaplaincy program, such as the one sponsored by the Association of Clinical Pastoral Education. He can also attend pastoral education courses and conferences offered in various centers and institutions throughout the country. And then, there is self-education through self-reflection while visiting the sick, and self-education through reading and studying the appropriate texts in both the secular and religious literature.

I have personally discovered that the greatest amount of learning in the area of visiting the sick comes from the last method. I have found that self-study and self-reflection have contributed to my inner growth in chaplaincy. In regard to self-study, there are of course many texts, beginning with Kübler-Ross' *On Death and Dying*, that are most valuable. But also, each religious tradition has texts that even though ancient can be applied to our ministry today and to the problems we are striving to overcome.

Within my own tradition, there are various Judaic texts that give some direction to the inquiring clergyman regarding the visiting of the sick. Some of the more ancient texts will give less direction than others, because it is difficult to transcribe their concepts of illness into modern thought and language. However, there are many useful texts. One of the most instructive passages on visiting the sick, and particularly those who have gone through a change in body image and self-image, is found in the sixteenth century text, *Shulchan Aruch*, by Joseph Karo. It is written in the book *Yoreh Deah*, Section 335:8, "One should not visit those suffering from diseases of the intestines, the eyes or the head; the intestines because of embarrassment, and the eyes and head because of a difficulty with speech. With those whose illness is severe and/or speech is difficult, one should stand in the antechamber and inquire about him, or offer whatever household or nursing help he may need, or sympathize with him and pray for him" (adapted from Chaim Demburg's translation).

This statement is adapted from the teaching of R. Jose ben Parta in R. Eliezer's name, which can be found in the Talmud *Nedarim* 41a. This talmudic section enumerates the above sicknesses as being excluded from the immediate need of visitation. As it is the diseases of the intestines, head, and neck that are specifically mentioned, the question must be asked, why are they mentioned? What are the problems involved in visiting patients with diseases of these areas of the body? I will address myself to the problem inherent in visiting that patient with intestinal or urological diseases.

The statement from the *Shulchan Aruch* speaks of the element of embarrassment that can be common to urological diseases and that can arise from a surgical procedure, which brings about a change in body image and self-image. The source of the embarrassment is the newness of the change brought about by the ileostomy or colostomy and in the way the patient sees himself and the way others will see him. "An ileostomy is a lifesaving measure, yet one cannot expect the patient to be grateful for its presence. Regardless of the severity of the inflammatory bowel disease and the toll it has taken, the ileostomy is an assault on the person's body image and self-esteem. Making a positive adaptive response to the stoma is a long and difficult task" (Watson, 1976, p. 428).

The same reaction is true for the colostomate. For him, that colostomy "can be the cause of untold mental and physical suffering" (Rowbotham, 1971, p. 4).

The change of body image comes with the patient's first view of the stoma and the attached appliance, which appears as a new "appendage" to the body. "Many patients are unprepared for the sight of the stoma" (Mahoney, 1978, p. 78). And there are, of course, the anxieties of touching it and caring for it. There is the concern of how others will see it, particularly one's spouse and loved ones. Change in self-image comes with learning to live with the odors emanating from the stoma, and with the noisy flatus sound. Both are "embarrassing and...a major cause for people avoiding social contacts" (Rowbotham, p. 6) and change in self-image also arises from the possibility of impotency, especially in males, and the fear of being unable to continue former professional, social, and recreational activities.

It is apparent that changes in physical appearance and function affect the emotional state of a person. Ostomy and prostate surgeries bring into question one's concept of self; the way one sees oneself through one's own eyes and the eyes of others. These questions are alluded to in the statement from the *Shulchan Aruch*, which gives direction to the visiting clergyman. To the patient, the clergyman represents the outside world that he will eventually have to reenter as a "changed" person. As such, the patient tests the visitor to see his reactions. I shall never forget visiting a gentleman who had had both a colostomy and an ileostomy the previous day. I had never met the man before. As I walked into the room, I was asked, "Would you like to see my scar?" Hesitantly, I replied, "O.K." He proceeded to lift up his gown and to show me his two stomas and his open wound from the laparotomy. The important part of this encounter was my verbal and physical reactions to what he had shown me. He was testing me and the outside world he would reenter. And since I was a clergyman, not dressed in doctor or nurse whites, I was even more representative of that "other" world. This testing occurs particularly during the period directly after surgery, a time when the patient needs the greatest amount of support and acceptance of who he is as a whole person, as a human being. This support must come from all the members of the helping team, with family, friends, and clergymen included. All must show acceptance.

The visiting clergyman should be aware of the odors, noises, and sights associated with the patient's operation. He must learn to accept what the patient is expressing and experiencing, for he must accept the patient as a whole person. As mentioned in the statement from the *Shulchan Aruch*, the inquiring clergyman should be cautious in entering the patient's room. While most hospitals today do not have an anteroom in which the visitor can stand and ask what he can do for the patient, the clergyman can walk into the room and be open for any verbal or nonverbal cues that tell him just how uncomfortable the patient might feel about the visit. The patient may not be ready to reveal himself, and the clergyman must respect him for this, or the patient might be ready but not express this readiness verbally. The clergyman must be sensitive to this cue also. The art of visiting must include the ability to end a conversation, either when the patient expresses this wish verbally, or through physical signs of exhaustion, pain, or discomfort. When a patient's self-image has been changed by surgery, the use of such knowledge will help the clergyman. Concern for another is shown when one refrains from placing the other in an embarrassing or uncomfortable situation.

Because visiting the sick is marked by respect for the patient, the clergyman should not draw attention to the patient's source of embarrassment unless the patient wants to discuss it. The clergyman should try to overcome his awareness of the intestinal or open-wound odors. The concern is for the person, and what gets in the way of relating to the person (the physical concomitants of illness and surgery) should be worked through and overcome by the visitor. Surely the patient should not be forced to engage in conversation if such conversation proves to be difficult or uncomfortable.

The statement in the *Shulchan Aruch* emphasizes that if the patient, despite the emotional and physical difficulties mentioned, wants to communicate with the clergyman or wants physical or spiritual care, advice, or counseling, the clergyman should be prepared for this. Notice should be taken that physical and practical considerations come first, and what we call counseling follows. Obtaining a glass of water, moving a tray, or positioning a pillow can be very important aspects of the clergyman's relationship with the patient who is suffering from a catastrophic illness that affects self-image. Such tasks in behalf of the patient's needs show the patient that people still care for him regardless of the way he looks, acts, or smells.

The visit is concluded by a blessing for God's mercy upon the patient. This last step is the goal of the clergyman's visit, according to the text as it is written in a commentary: "He who visits and does not request mercy upon the sick, it is as if he did not visit at all." This blessing shows the patient that in spite of his condition and the way he might see himself, the community and God will not abandon him. As the clergyman gives his presence out of his care for the whole person, so too will the community and God.

As a member of the healing team, the clergyman is most vital. He represents a community outside the hospital that cares for the patient as a whole person. The clergyman can make significant contributions to the patient's healing process because he understands that process and the role he plays in its function. It has been shown that those patients "who did best were those whose period of adjustment had been strongly supported by those persons who were most important to them" (Prudden, 1971, p. 18). Then the task of each clergyman is to learn how to show that support.

References

Mahoney, J.M..: What you should know about ostomies. *Nursing 78, 8* (5):428, May, 1978.
Prudden, J.F.: Psychological problems following ileostomy and colostomy. In *Rehabilitation of the Patient with Colostomy*. American Cancer Society, 1971, p. 18.
Rowbotham, J.L.: Colostomy problems—Dietary and colostomy management. In *Rehabilitation of the Patient with Colostomy*. American Cancer Society, 1971, p. 4.
Watson, P.G., Wood, R.Y., Wechsler, N.L., and Christensen, L.: Comprehensive care of the ileostomy patient. *Nursing Clinics of North America, 11* (3):428, September, 1976.

Chapter 4

CARING — THE HEART OF OSTOMY NURSING

Mary A. Csensits

As an enterostomal therapist, I help patients adjust to changes in body functions. I care for and help the ostomate, a person with a surgically created and permanent abdominal opening for the elimination of excreta. The needs of these patients go far beyond physical requirements. It is the aim of the enterostomal therapist to aid in rehabilitation — to instruct patients about adjustments in daily living, including diet, exercise, occupation, and individual hygienic techniques. Our goal is to return patients to a full, happy, productive life. My professional experiences have provided me with information and insights that can diminish the myth and mystery from the "hole in the side" and remove some of the stigma patients have had to endure.

The ileal conduit is the most frequently performed permanent urinary diversion with an external stoma. In this procedure, the surgeon isolates a 15 to 17.5 cm (6 to 8 inches) piece of ileum and retains the mesentery to maintain blood supply. The ureters are anastomosed to the ileal segment, then the proximal end is closed and the distal end is brought through the abdominal wall and secured to the skin as a mature stoma. It is now a diversion before it reaches the bladder. The isolated length of ileum acts as a conduit (urine flows from the kidneys through the ureters and ileal loop directly to the external urinary appliance without any internal urine storage). A permanent appliance on the outside of the body takes over for a defunct bladder.

Case Illustration

My patient, Louis, is a 53-year-old male who was admitted with a diagnosis of adenocarcinoma of the prostate and a Grade III invasive transitional cell carcinoma of the urinary bladder. He was scheduled to have an ileal conduit. The attending surgeon introduced the idea of surgery and talked with the patient about his cancer and the need for care. Upon the request of the urologist, I met Louis a day after his admission.

After my first meeting with Louis I saw him on a daily basis preoperatively and clarified aspects of future care in reference to his ileal conduit. I was able to discuss the diagnosis openly with the patient. However, when Louis was given the option of viewing the type of appliance that he would wear the rest of his life, he stated that he was not interested. Then it appeared more meaningful to talk with the patient about eliminating the cause of his trouble and about how the planned surgery was designed to do that. In this period, I wanted him to develop feelings of trust as an important basis in my care for him. Trust does not arise automatically; it must be a part of the history or a particular relationship or be earned. Once earned, it must be maintained.

When Louis was told about his cancer and the need for a change in his body image because of the ileal conduit, he exhibited a certain amount of fear and anxiety. Some of the emotional feelings and strain he encountered stemmed from the fact that among his earliest accomplishments in life was control of urination, a function bound by strong emotional components. Losing control implied a return to infant life and subsequent loss of self-esteem. The mutilative surgery frightened him; no longer would he come close to society's idea of the perfect body. He felt that his physical appearance would be robbed of its integrity. He would not be confronted with just a scar, but an opening from which he would express his uncontrolled urine. Louis entertained all these ideas and decided the price would be a small one to pay for his life.

He was also concerned about sexual activity after the operation. Although many statistics relative to postsurgery impotence are available, I have found it better to give the patient general information. In attempting to do research in this area, I have found it difficult to find any completely helpful guide. Therefore, I have come to a conclusion prompted by answers I have received in the past: "To each his own." Current concepts of acceptable sexual techniques make it possible for a large number of people to enjoy a satisfactory sex life. The ostomate must be assured that the stoma is not easily "squished" or smothered. There is no, or negligible, risk of stoma injury during sexual intercourse. An eager and understanding sex partner is not inhibited by a stoma and does not permit its presence to interfere with the pleasure that has been aroused by a desirable partner.

People have different attitudes about sex based on education, religion, and personality. I told Louis about a single girl, an ostomate, who never told her prospective bed partner ahead of time about her surgery because she never intended to see him again. If the surgery and the equipment are unacceptable to his mate, the mate's maturity and true love should be questioned, not the ostomate's physical abilities. I told Louis that perhaps sex is 90 percent in the head and 10 percent below the waist. When actual impotence has resulted, a penile implant or alternative methods of sexual satisfaction may be explored.

I spent a great amount of time with Louis prior to his radical surgery. I helped him move toward his goal during this emotional crisis. He found himself in a situation he really did not want to accept. He dreaded the time he would have to spend in the intensive care unit. I had designs to help Louis through this life crisis. I accepted my patient during his stressful preoperative period and wanted to share and be a great part of his care, along with his physicians and the nursing staff. While it is true that ostomy patients have specialized nursing needs, we know that the success we have had is primarily due to basic nursing techniques. High quality of care is based on sound judgment, keen observation, emotional support, and in-depth teaching. The patient's wife is involved in the care whenever possible, and she was involved in Louis' case. I felt that we had a coordinated and cooperative team effort and that my patient was ready for surgery.

Every patient goes through four phases of recovery following an accident, illness, or results of a function, whether a paraplegic, hemiplegic, or an ostomate. Every phase requires a period of time. The spouse and family especially must help and aid the patient get through these phases:

A. *First Phase*: The Shock Phase. This is the period of psychological impact patients do not remember after surgery. A lot of support is required.

B. *Second Phase*: The Defensive Retreat Phase. The patient avoids reality. There is wishful thinking, denial, or repression of his actual condition.

C. *Third Phase*: Phase of Acknowledgment. The individual faces the realities of his crisis, then enters a period of depression, apathy, agitation, bitterness, and high anxiety.

D. *Fourth Phase*: Period of Adaptation. The patient actively copes with the situation in a constructive manner. He adopts the adjustments that are necessary.

I saw Louis early on the day his surgery was scheduled. He had had his preoperative medication but was not sleeping. He acknowledged my presence and appeared to be in good spirits. He made some incidental remark about his postoperative course, projecting the time that he would be out of bed and on the road to recovery. I encouraged him and wanted him to attain his optimal state of health and fulfillment after surgery. The patient was taken to the operating room.

It is my routine to see patients immediately after surgery in the recovery room. This also gives me the opportunity to speak to the nursing staff and to reinforce aspects of care necessary for scientific nursing of the ostomate. The patient was doing well from a surgical point of view, and the temporary appliance over his stoma and attached to straight drainage revealed no complications. After discharge from the recovery room, the patient was admitted to the intensive care unit and remained there for a brief period. Then, he was transferred to a regular surgical nursing unit.

Louis' postoperative course was uneventful. I attributed this to the continued individualized nursing care, including skilled physical nursing care and emotional support afforded by all caregivers. I explored my own attitudes and any negative feelings that I had about a stoma. I exercised my own emotional support system to the utmost. I emphasized the need for other rehabilitation rather than just the stoma.

Gradually, the patient developed an awareness of his stoma and also realized that a private function was now in evidence. To accomplish the latter, much verbalization must be carried out in reference to what the stoma looks like, what its function is, and the need for the external appliance. It was obvious that the stoma was a disadvantage, but at this time the patient did not have too much difficulty coping with the external appliance that contained the urine. The patient's physical involvement in the application of his permanent appliance was encouraged daily, and he became adept within a short period of time. After this, the patient's wife was also instructed in the care of the ostomy. The visiting nurse was introduced to the patient and his wife, and arrangements were made for her to aid in a smooth transition from hospital to home.

During the patient's hospitalization, we provided him with information covering the emotional, physical, cultural, and social aspects of life with an ostomy. The patient was discharged ten days after surgery. To quote an observation by a student nurse in her evaluation of this patient, "The patient seems to fully understand the care necessary and seems confident." We all felt Louis acknowledged his ostomy as a therapeutic measure. I do think he proved all observations to be valid because he took a nurse in his arms without warning and said, "Let's dance!" They danced a few steps and he was ready to leave the hospital.

What is caring? Caring is our regard for the health, happiness, and comfort of the patient. Care is concern for the disease process and the results of the treatment on the whole person. We care for persons in all phases of illness. It is a caring until death. It is our aim to make the management of dying more sensible and compassionate.

Care should be directed at total pain, including physical, mental, social, and spiritual pain. Treatment programs should be directed at symptoms, pain, and diseases that deprive the patient of strength for living. It is the caregiver's responsibility to help the dying person to live until the moment of death.

Dying and death must not be ignored. We must create an awareness and talk about them. Two million Americans are dying each year, and more than 90 percent die in institutions. Because of scientific advances, man rarely dies in the comfort of his own home, surrounded by family and friends gathered to pay their last respects. He is comforted by an oxygen tank, tubes in every natural and surgically made orifice, and busy hospital personnel intent on carrying out the physician's orders.

Seventy-five years ago, there was no need for a dying oriented nurse. Patients died in the settings in which they had spent their lives. Fortunately, the medical professions realize that the needs of those who cannot be saved should be met.

Before we are able to understand the needs of the dying, we must develop a personal philosophy of death and dying and expose ourselves to this experience. We must examine our attitude toward death and understand the basic reactions to dying. There is a simple proposition in life: love first, know second. If this is kept in the right order, the care of these patients becomes simplified. When we have some concept of what they are experiencing while we listen, watch, and care for them, then the practical problems can be handled on an individual level with our own creative powers. Working through feelings may be the most important yet difficult process to improved nursing care. The phrases we use when we have empathy are not important. We need not learn a verbal approach; the proper expressions will come.

When Louis was readmitted to the hospital a little more than two months later, we had another opportunity to care for him. He was admitted because of complaints in his lower abdominal area and rectal discomfort. According to the patient's statement, he was taking different medications: to treat an ulcer, to control his pain, and to maintain bowel function. He was admitted under the care of the urologists. After examination and a blood workup, Louis was referred to the general surgeons. Because of apparent peritonitis and because the patient's condition was worsening, an exploratory laparotomy was performed by the general surgeon with his urologist assisting.

Upon entrance into the peritoneal cavity, a large amount of white exudate was found throughout the serosal surface of the intestine and omentum. A perforated duodenal ulcer was closed and there was a serosal patch of impending perforation of the descending colon. He had a closure of the patch in that area; and a diverting distal transverse colostomy and a decompressing jejunostomy were performed. The patient returned from the operating room with an appliance over his ileal conduit and colostomy. A sump drain was inserted into the site of the jejunostomy. The ileal conduit was functioning well.

Caring for Louis at this time was not easy. Listed here are some of the statements on his chart, revealing the thoughts of members of the caregiving team:

"Is acutely ill, has fever and sepsis."
"Pouches changed because of leakage."
"Proximal loop of the colostomy irrigated."
"The patient looks weaker."

"I don't know if our efforts in encouraging him will help; he is so depressed."
"Patient is drinking Gatorade."
"The patient is having a personality change."
"He is alert, but weak. Cooperative."
"Condition is worsening. Is vomiting. Is hallucinating."
"Picking at things in the air."
"Taking Gatorade. The problem with the duodenal drainage was one mainly of nutrition."
"Was out of bed. The patient does not look bad."
"Weak and lethargic. Had chills. Was seen by the rehab nurse."
"Looks surprisingly well in spite of his problems. Fever 101°."
"Possible subphrenic collection or a septic CVP catheter."
"Developed a fistula through the lower portion of his abdominal wound."
"Successfully placed a tube into the duodenum beyond the fistula."
"Draining frankly purulent material through lower portion of his incision."
"Now wearing three plastic pouches."
"Responds to questions. Rational and talking. Is in better spirits."
"Seems a bit clearer. Patient is alert, joking. Still taking Gatorade."

Six weeks later, the patient was able to witness the wedding of his son; it took place in the patient's semiprivate room, and a promise by his son was fulfilled. The minister, a friend who saw the patient quite often and gave sensitive, tender support, performed the ceremony. In the process of the patient's illness, the family and patient grew and gave support to each other.

Then care continued with further observations noted in the chart:

"Looks weaker; the patient was encouraged; has chills; is talkative and interested in his care."
"The patient is slowly beginning to express his feelings about his condition and the length of time he has been ill. He notes the size of his arms and makes general remarks about his recovery."

The patient lost about one-third of his body weight. His temperature was 102° and a blood culture was done. The organism pseudomonas aeruginosa was identified. To say the least, it had become a horrifying and escalating situation.

I thought my patient was dying, but it was difficult to talk with Louis about death. I waited for cues from him, but he did not seek me out. On one occasion, I distinctly recall that he said to me, "They will take me home in a pine box." Viewing his frail body, I felt the patient was probably correct. I assured him that I would continue to do all that was possible to make him comfortable, but avoided any false assurances. I tried not to weep with him but allowed him to know that I realized he was in a difficult situation and that I felt for him. Oral care seemed to be an important activity to make him comfortable. Seeking the aid of another nurse to help me put him in a better sitting position in order to facilitate his breathing was another factor in making him comfortable.

Caring for Louis was becoming a long and frightening experience. I am sure he realized from his physical signs that the situation was grave. He was concerned about himself. But was it really helpful to tell him how he was progressing? On another occasion, he asked me, "When am I going to get better?" I thought Louis was dying by degrees, but I could in no way create for him an awareness of his impending death. I listened and watched and let him indicate when he wanted more information. His way of handling the situation was denial. I encouraged him not to give up his fight.

The scientific nursing problems involved in a situation where a patient wears three plastic pouches become complex. The staff, especially young nurses, found working with such a patient depressing. Their nursing management was involved and time consuming. But the power of the young dedicated nurse who uses her education well should not be underestimated. One particular neophyte who was caring for Louis was free to make her own nursing assessments, and she planned care accordingly. She was kind and gentle. I saw her developing her clinical expertise, and our patient received much benefit from her skills. On many occasions, Louis would tell me how he appreciated the care given by one nurse as compared with that given by another. He made observations about his depressed and distressed state and about the material and human aspects of his care, and even mentioned the kiss on the forehead given by one nurse. I think Louis had confidence and trust in the people who provided his care. Most of the nurses realized that he was a challenge. They attempted to control his pain because they realized that when he ate and slept better, his anxiety was greatly reduced.

There were periods of heavy distress for the nurses also and a need to support one another and to be sensitive to their own emotional needs. I spent time with the nursing staff and wanted them to share my particular skills and concerns.

When I thought things were going well, they began to fall apart. The patient's wife was asking me, "How long can I take this?" She complained about the nurses, and the staff began to complain about situations they noticed in regard to Louis' family.

The patient's condition did not change much. This was the crux of the matter. He again spiked a fever and was very depressed. He now weighed 113 pounds. His blood culture this time identified the Klebsiella oxytoca organism. My role as an enterostomal therapist, nurse, teacher, friend, and counselor changed to that of coordinator. After listening to all the complaints and laments from the people involved in his care, I felt that I must do something to remedy the worsening situation. I did not know exactly where to begin or what to do; I felt hopeless.

After a great deal of thought, I made a plan. I saw Roberta, the patient's wife, spoke to the nurse who works in the admitting department, and then contacted the attending surgeons about transferring the patient to a private room. Everyone involved felt this would be a good idea. I also obtained the information that if a patient needed a private room because of medical reasons, a written note from the attending surgeon would convince Blue Cross–Blue Shield to pick up its cost. I was attempting to conserve finances as well as Louis' strength.

The change to a private room was a good idea. The patient seemed to get more rest, but his condition did not change over any given period of time. On one occasion, I attempted to extract some feelings from Louis: "Louis, I guess you are pretty tired of the whole situation."

He looked at me and said, "You bet I am, Ginger." He went on to say, "How about the irrigations—do you think they are still needed?"

Louis stabilized and was discharged. His weight at the time of discharge was 106 pounds. His colostomy and ileal conduit were working well, and his oral intake was acceptable.

Louis continues his fight; he worries about himself and his condition, but he never appears resigned to his fate. Maybe he did not want to experience the loss of future sense. When this is lost, it is particularly traumatic and the ego can find no adequate way to cope with the stress. I had no plans to change his mind. His frail body and determined mind go on living. We will continue to give him the best of care. He knows that we are concerned about his feelings. He needs comfort, courage, and hope. We will continue to help Louis achieve inner growth, despite his physical decline.

Bibliography

Barckley, V.: What can I say to the cancer patient? *Nursing Outlook,* 6:316-318, June, 1958.
Barckley, V.: Enough time for good nursing. *Nursing Outlook,* 12:44-48, April, 1964.
Craytor, J.K.: Talking with persons who have cancer. *American Journal of Nursing,* 69 (4):744-748, 1969.
Earle, A.M., Argondizzo, N.T., and Kutscher, A.H. (Eds.): *The Nurse as Caregiver for the Terminal Patient and His Family.* New York, Columbia University Press, 1976.
Fox, J.E.: Reflections on cancer nursing. *American Journal of Nursing,* 66 (6):1317-1319.
Verwoerdt, A.: Communication with the fatally ill. *Southern Medical Journal,* 57:787-795, 1964.

Chapter 5

TREATMENT OF THE CANCER PATIENT BY THE PRIMARY CARE PHYSICIAN

HYMAN L. MUSLIN AND SUSAN P. LEVINE

THE attending physician who is to be the cancer patient's caregiver clearly has a multitude of concerns relating to the patient's physiologic welfare. We are here concerned with an attempt to delineate the psychosocial variables in the patient and in the physician that will be of assistance in the management of the patient and perhaps be of some service to the physician. It is, of course, no small task to enter into the life space of the patient ill with cancer and to offer company, sympathy, and even empathy. Therefore, it often seems necessary to request a psychiatric consultation in an attempt to relieve oneself of the burden of alleviating the depression or anxiety so often exhibited by a cancer patient. Unfortunately, these psychiatric consultations are often a one-interview experience for the patient and cannot be followed up because of the usual situation in which there are only a fixed number of liaison psychiatrists in the ordinary hospital staff. Thus, the psychiatrist interviews, writes attitude orders, and may meet with the attending physician once to agree with the diagnosis of depression, to suggest a minor tranquilizer or an antidepressant, and even to advise that more visits be made by the family. At this point, the psychiatrist withdraws and in effect gives license to the attending physician to imitate his model of withdrawal.

The situation must be faced more directly; in fact, there is an understandable but not acceptable reaction of the physician to the cancer patient, and it is often a reaction of rejection. The issue surrounds the reaction on the part of physicians to the treatment of someone who is most likely to die while under treatment. We ask of our physicians that they empathize in all cases with the total patient.

In the case of the cancer patient, we are asking physicians to vicariously introspect, to identify with the feelings of a dying person, a person who is in a chronic mourning state and who is living through the permanent separation from life. While these features of the permanent separation may be denied for a long while by the physician, there is, to be sure, a constant underlying awareness (preconscious) of the death knell in the patient's surrounding. The physican's capacity for empathy is interfered with by the usual avoidances and denials surrounding death and the dying manifest in interpersonal encounters between patient and physician, often as a rejection of the total patient, and replaced by behavior ranging from overemphasis on the physiologic to complete avoidance of the patient to hostility reactions to the patient. Many other varieties of this rejection behavior can be seen, including the substitution of psychological mottos for understanding of people, as for example in the motto, "Disclosure of all pertinent information is *the* only approach to cancer patients," or "Withholding of all (as much as one can) information is the most acceptable approach in the communication of cancer patients." These mottos can serve, and usually do, as a resistance to the necessary interaction with cancer patients, since it seems clear that the complex psychological reactions to cancer and impending death must, of course, be carefully assessed and one's communication, as in all serious interpersonal behavior, is to be based on careful observation of the individual's behavior: What one tells is a function of what one observes. And so we are left with the usual observations that both physician and patient often have a great deal of difficulty in relating to one another when the patient's diagnosis of cancer becomes apparent. We have also stated that much of this difficulty is a manifestation of the usual uneasiness that reflects the physician's empathic difficulties in dealing with the patient who is close to death.

The physician of the cancer patient, to be effective, cannot without special experiences be expected to perform the empathic work required to appreciate and be of service in maintaining psychological equilibrium. The training in observation and collating of the behavior and emotional state of physiologically sick patients is usually lacking in most of our hospitals. While some medical schools highlight observations of behavior as a value, these emphases will not be helpful to the practitioner in oncology unless he or she obtains special support and encouragement to utilize the skills and techniques of psychiatry. The answer rests with a psychiatry department, which can become involved in an ongoing teaching and service relationship. So a model for data gathering, a model of data collating, and finally an emphasis on therapy modalities and the evolving of a treatment plan — all these approaches should be used in the training of the physician on the wards.

Still another major variable in the psychological treatment of the patient is the physician's usual conflicts to which we have alluded — the complex processes stirred up in the physician attending a patient who is chronically ill and commonly fatally ill.

We are asking a great deal of our primary care physicians when we ask that they should maintain an optimal distance so as to care for the cancer patient. A physician's capacity for empathy is strained a great deal when dealing with the fatally ill. The nature of the strain is the anxiety and guilt evoked by witnessing a person known to be dying or close to dying while under one's care. It certainly is true that veteran observers of cancer patients and other patients fatally ill do master their subjective reactions and become more helpful over time. However, many reactions, as we have noted, represent avoidances, denials, and a variety of either unhelpful or negative reactions *since* what occurs to the physician of the cancer patient is the stimulation of his or her buried fears over the dying process. Ordinarily, the physician has adjusted to death but has not observed, in himself or herself, and appreciated the fantasies that make dying and death painful or frightening. Thus, whatever untoward or fearful responses are evoked in the care of a cancer patient are ordinarily shunned and replaced by defenses that will militate against attention to the emotional needs of the patient. To be empathic requires that our physicians be removed from their narcissistic preoccupation, i.e. a physician caring for any patient is at a loss if his own welfare is at stake, when the physician is also seeking sustenance or deliverance from a frightening scene.

The Body of Skills and Knowledge

The ideal approach to the patient is based on a model of careful observation of the patient's total behavior, which then allows for judicious management in the attempts to maintain the patient's equilibrium. These observations include attention to the patient's verbal and nonverbal behavior in a serious attempt to evaluate the patient's psychic equilibrium. Literally, it means that the behaviors are as carefully assessed, as is the acid-base balance or the x-ray reports. When the physician adopts this model of careful observations and study of behavior, his mission changes from the task of responding intuitively to the more helpful mode of listening, observing, and studying the behavior. From this data base one *can* make the comments that are needed, or also one can decide that comments are not needed.

These observations need to be placed into a framework that will assist the physician in assessing the patient's current psychological status. The physician must first note and appraise the frank signs of psychological disequilibrium. These are the manifestations of frank major anxiety, overt intense depressive reactions, and also major regressive responses including disorganized or fragmented behavior. These manifestations are to be distinguished from modal anxiety or modal depressions, which are not signs of disequilibrium but behavior responses to being ill. A patient in mourning due to the overt or covert knowledge of cancer is not in disequilibrium. Likewise, the eruption of anxiety from time to time is a sign of the usual reaction to the knowledge of impending death. A response of regressive behavior is a common reaction to cancer and death, and if it consists of more passivity and receptivity is often an adaptative response to being seriously ill. The chronic anxiety state, the state of unremitting depression with major loss of self-esteem, and the vegetative signs of depression are the data that indicate frank disequilibrium and represent a need for therapeutic intervention. We have also noted that a major regression is a further sign of disequilibrium; we are referring to the behavior of disorganization, of infantile states, and the like. Thus, the first judgment to be made is whether or not the patient is in disequilibrium or not.

The next task is to attempt to recognize the manner in which the patient is responding to the stress of the illness. The attempts to resolve the stress of the illness take place by way of shifts in the psychic apparatus so that the patient undergoes changes in his or her ego defenses, self system, and superego. The defenses are mechanisms that serve to maintain repression of the drives arising for immediate discharge. These mechanisms are manifest as, for example, in the behavior of denial, an attempt to shun or avoid reality ("my tumor is smaller today"). Another common defense that is enacted is the defense of projection, the externalization of different aspects of the psychic apparatus. Other familiar mechanisms are displacement (substitution of one object of concern or anger for another), regression (a change to an earlier form of functioning), repression (psychic forgetting), reaction formation (adoption of attitudes which are the opposite of the emerging drive, sweetness replacing sadism), and identification (as seen in the patient emulating the physician).

These defenses represent valuable methods of maintaining equilibrium but at times, carried to an extreme, they are maladaptive or even interfere with the testing with reality. A patient may deny for too long a time the existence of a lump in her breast with tragic consequences; the denial of illness at times becomes so pronounced that it represents a major break with reality and constitutes a need for intervention. Thus a patient operating to deny reality may become euphoric and grandiosely wish for discharge while undergoing antimetabolite therapy for a lymphoma.

Another major psychological change is in the patient's self-system, which represents the patient's perceptions of his entire soma and psyche and the self-regard (narcissism). There is ordinarily a change in one's self-regard and perceptions of oneself. The acceptance of patienthood implies that a person can live comfortably in the role of one who is cared for and implies that no significant loss of self-esteem take place. Often, there is a loss in self-regard, one of the features of depression, and sometimes a massive loss of narcissism takes place, representing a need for intervention to protect against suicide.

Next, it is important to evaluate the changes in the patient's superego, which represents both the patient's moral values (conscience, taboos, prohibitions) and ideals (aspirations, goals for oneself). Ordinarily, if a patient's behavior does not transgress the moral codes, he does not experience *guilt*. Also, if he lives up to his ideals, there will be no experience of *shame* or feelings of inferiority. Any casual observer of a pool of cancer patients knows that guilt feelings (I've been bad; I've hurt my family; I caused my cancer) and shame feelings (I'm not a man any more; don't bother with me) are unfortunately common. Perhaps the ideal superego response is a relaxation of moral codes and standards so that one can tolerate the emerging dependency and aggression without guilt or shame.

Finally, the physician needs to judge the overall adaptation to the environment by the patient. Adaptation refers to the mastery of the environment and thus is a reflection of the integrity of the defenses, the self-system changes and the other transformations of the psychic apparatus. A successful adaptation may come about, therefore, with a moderate amount of denial of the seriousness of the illness or a displacement and projection with changes in the self and a transformation of the conscience.

The relationship the patient makes with the physician needs to be considered separately since it represents one of the major factors in the treatment of any patient with any illness. One facet of the relationship represents the reality-based feature of the expert-client interaction — the expert doctor giving advice, performing a procedure, or instructing the patient. Another facet of the interaction represents times, situations or therapies when the doctor and patient form an alliance to work on a common problem, such as is the case with a patient taking medication and reporting effects, i.e. the patient and physician are allying themselves in a common effort. Another aspect of the relationship is the transference the patient makes onto the physician of old and fantasied aspirations and gratifications from the significant figures and interactions of infancy and childhood. The physician in fantasy is experienced as the latter-day representatives of one's mother, father, brother, or sister and therefore is respected, feared, cherished, or hated. Not only is it important to recognize these intricacies of the physician–patient relationship in each interaction with each patient, but also it is one of the major management issues in patients. Every patient requires a specialized interaction based on the observable behavior that delineates the patient's need of the doctor as an ally, as comforter, as expert, or even as taskmaster.

The Training-Learning Issues

An approach to the learning of the matters of observation, collating, and management should take the form of seminars and individual supervision. Seminars are needed on observation and collating that consist of poring over videotaped diagnostic interviews so that the essential behaviors can be isolated. Here, one can demonstrate the behaviors of all kinds, while giving the necessary theoretical information. In this setting, one can also demonstrate the organizing of the behavior so as to formulate a management plan.

Also, one can demonstrate with videotaped interviews an approach to the management of a patient who demonstrates a particular problem.

The next learning phase consists of supervision of one or several physicians who report on a particular patient they are managing. The supervisor, ordinarily a psychiatrist (or a nonpsychiatric physician who has had the necessary experience and training), goes over the data and points out the interventions required or the missed observations. It is extremely valuable to obtain a videotape or audiotape of the actual interaction between the physician and the patient. At times it is only when the physician sees himself with the patient that some vital aspect of the interaction can come to light. The setting may vary, but it is helpful for the teaching to take place on the wards, in medicine and surgery.

The Model

The model of the caregiver of the cancer patient is that of the physician as *menschenkenner*, the physician who functions as diagnostician of the emotional equilibrium and thus the emotional needs of the patient. This physician is also to initiate a plan of psychological management that may range from simple institution of a special relationship, e.g. of the alliance model of relatedness, the relationship based on being a supporting parent, to manipulation of the environment in a special manner that suits the patient's needs. The physician is also to be available and helpful in the special therapeutic needs of the family, i.e. the physician is to be alert to the needs of the family for education, ventilation, and support.

Management Modes

The psychosocial management of patients must deal with issues that are, at times, clearly psychological but also, at times, clearly environmental. All psychological approaches to the emotional aspects of the cancer patient are in the direction of support and maintenance of psychological equilibrium. The actual technique utilized will come out of the initial attempts to observe and collate the behavior of the patient.

Supportive psychotherapy encompasses a variety of techniques to initiate and maintain psychosocial behavior. One such important measure is the specific use of the physician–patient relationship for support. The physician must in this category of techniques be careful in the assessment of the relationship that will best provide support for this patient at this time. Thus, for one cancer patient in whom the data demonstrate that the patient is frightened, experiencing fragility, and desperately requesting attention and reassurance, the physician clearly is called on to be the omniscient, nurturing parent–surrogate whom the patient needs for relief of the fear. In another patient in whom the data reveal a person uneasy with anxiety and shame, the physician may utilize the alliance model and maintain a friendly air with equanimity displayed in his posture to the patient. Another relationship model is necessary when a patient is markedly regressed and needs a great deal of structure; the patient is alternately demanding of interest but also obdurate and, at times, unable to cooperate with the physician and staff. Here the posture of the physician needs to become that of the authority figure who details the behavior required with firmness and even command. An important principle in the intelligent utilization of the relationship is that the relationship must be a reflection of the current behavior and needs of the patient; a patient two days postoperation is a different person from the same patient ten days after surgery, and thus the relationship must change accordingly. A patient anxious about the diagnosis of the lesion will need a different approach from the same patient after the diagnosis is known. A special note must be made about the needs manifest throughout all forms of relationship for the need to express affects and all behaviors within the physician–patient interaction. At times, the physician must be available to the patient for ventilation and abreaction of affects; the patient needs to cry, to rage, and to mourn. The physician in these situations needs to be an available friend, without interventions, who simply recognizes and accepts the meaningful discharge of affects.

Another supportive measure is the specific support of defenses and the self-system. In the case of a patient whose equilibrium is maintained by *denial*, the physician is called on to support this defense. The physician does not challenge or threaten the defense within certain clear-cut bounds. A patient's breeziness or avoidance of certain topics is to be accepted and even entered into; however, the denial cannot be accepted if it interferes with treatment, surgery, and so forth. A vital aspect of support is the recognition of the patient's need for esteem, which is also a part of the relationship required to maintain equilibrium.

A therapeutic measure that is supportive is the organization of the environment in a way that is most helpful to the particular patient. So it is that one patient is in need of a homey atmosphere with flowers, visitors, friendliness, and music, whereas another patient needs to identify with the staff and to be given clinical tasks, books to read, and information about the illness to promote intellectualization and the like.

At times, in those patients in whom the defenses are inimical to the overall equilibrium and who are accessible enough to form a workable relationship, the physician may be called upon to confront the patient with the special defense or conflict the data reveal. The physician focuses on giving the patient insight into the distressing affect or defenses to reinstitute equilibrium. Insight here is confined to becoming aware, observing a defense or affect and in this manner neutralizing this defense. In actual practice, a patient who is exhibiting behavior that is inimical to his or her progress must be confronted in an attempt to inhibit the behavior and help the patient see the behavior in action and isolate the defense, acting out, or other distressing behavior. As in all psychotherapy activities, the patient in this activity learns the techniques of observing by identifying with the physician; it is in effect a stimulus to intellectualization.

The use of antianxiety and antidepressant drugs is an important measure in the treatment of emotional disturbance, as is the judicious use of hypnotics for sleep disturbances. These drugs can never and should never be used to replace the physician–patient interaction but may be helpful in alleviating anxiety and depression.

The anxiety that is manifest ordinarily can best be treated by diazepam (Valium®) or chlordiazepoxide (Librium®). Tranquilizers are not to be used like digitalis or insulin; they should be used if there is anxiety but for one or two or three times and then reevaluated the following day and not reordered for weeks at a time without monitoring. An anxiety attack on one occasion does not indicate a six-month regimen on a tranquilizer without monitoring.

These considerations also pertain to the use of antidepressants but in a different manner. The use of antidepressants is to be confined to relief of the vegetative signs of depression, essentially psychomotor retardation, anorexia, sleep disturbance. There is also an alleviation of the mood disturbance of sadness so that relief from depression is obtained with these compounds. The treatment with antidepressants, imipramine or amitryptyline, involves a one- to three-week latency time when the compounds build up concentration and then an indeterminate time when the symptoms diminish and then another time period for prevention (six months to several years). Relief of anxiety and relief of the symptoms of depression, especially loss of self-esteem, are important measures to undertake. We personally do not feel that cancer patients should suffer with the psychic pain of fear or loss of esteem. Thus, pharmacotherapy may be an important feature of any program of psychotherapy with cancer patients.

The use of hypnotics is also important in maintaining equilibrium. The physician must be careful to use nonbarbiturates and safe compounds that do not interfere with normal sleep (REM) patterns.

The Setting

The physician who manages the emotional problems of his patients on the wards must perform the therapeutic work in a variety of settings and without the appointments and time frames and all the other trappings that go with ordinary outpatient practice. The work of observing patients' moods and behaviors must go on, at times, during the initial history and physical examination. At times, the observing work must go on during ward rounds or during a treatment procedure. The actual psychotherapeutic interaction sometimes goes on while starting an I.V. or while taking a blood sample. Thus it is that each contact with each patient in any setting is a psychotherapeutic encounter, sometimes from a diagnostic point of view. At times, the physician can and must see the patient in the office to engage in an important dialogue centering around a special difficulty that will require thirty-five to forty minutes of unimpeded work. However, there is a great deal of work that can be accomplished during ward rounds — during a brief encounter on the wards while performing a procedure. Thus, a diagnosis of emotional needs may be established during a history-taking session, and other times of observation and the actual psychological treatment may be carried out during ward rounds, occasional office visits, or spontaneous meetings in treatment rooms.

In closing, three clinical examples are included to illustrate how psychiatric principles may be applied in the medical situation to either diagnose or manage a clinical problem. The first case represents a common diagnostic problem — that of severe depression occurring during a terminal illness.

> *Case 1.* The patient was a fifty-two-year-old man who was under treatment for a stage IV lymphoma. The patient had married a younger woman six months previously and had developed symptoms of his lymphoma three months previously. The lymphoma was poorly responsive to chemotherapy, and the patient was rapidly losing ground. On the basis of reading he had done on his own, which indicated that patients may live many years with lymphoma, the patient maintained an optimistic outlook that became increasingly unrealistic in the light of his physical decline. The patient began to wonder how long he had to live, and bluntly put this question to his doctor. The answer he obtained, according to him, was "a year or less." Following this, he became severely depressed and embittered toward his doctor and the hospital and expressed anger at having been given a death sentence. His depressive thoughts focused on feelings of generalized weakness and weakness of his legs and inability to work or to provide for his new wife. "I feel like I am not really a man," he said. In describing an incident in which he had collapsed while trying to walk, the patient said, "I couldn't help it. It wasn't my fault." He resisted efforts to send him home, although he also complained about being kept in the hospital so long. His behavior on the ward was depressed and hostile, and evoked an avoidance reaction on the part of the staff.

In our opinion, the critical observations in this vignette are that (1) the patient engineered his own death sentence so that he might use it for a psychological purpose; (2) he denied responsibility for his weakness, suggesting guilt over unconscious wishes to be relieved of his obligations as a man; and (3) weakness from his lymphoma was equated in his mind with not being adequate as a man. We infer from this that the patient's sudden depression was due to wishes, unacceptable to his superego and to his narcissistic self, to be relieved of the necessity to perform as a man. Supportive treatment for this patient, therefore, included the explicit assurance from his physician that his weakness (impotence) was caused by his disease and that he should not be expected to function as a healthy man.

The issue of whether or not to "tell" the diagnosis of cancer is raised by the following case:

> *Case 2.* A man in his early sixties was referred because of extreme chronic anxiety and obsessive preoccupation with his ileostomy. The patient had

been operated on for carcinoma of the colon eleven years previously, and although he tended to be anxious in general, had had no episodes of gross psychological disequilibrium in the interim, knowing only that he had had a "mass tumor" removed. One year prior to our interview the patient developed symptoms of a second primary in his colon, and before his colectomy he was told, without his asking, that he had a cancer and that he had had a cancer eleven years previously. The patient reacted to this information with intense anxiety and was obsessively preoccupied with cancer from then on. His preoccupation with his poorly healed ileostomy was seen to be a displacement of his fear that the cancer had recurred in the stoma.

The critical observations in this case are that the patient had done relatively well psychologically for a long period of time with the diagnosis of "mass tumor," that the patient had not asked to be told whether or not he had cancer, and that once he had been given the word *cancer* he was never able to adapt to it. Despite the persuasive case that can be made for full disclosure of all medical information to the patient, we feel that this case demonstrates that there are some patients who should never be told that they have cancer, and the decision whether to tell or not depends on an assessment of the patient's capacity to tolerate the word *cancer* and all that that diagnosis implies. Frequently, patients become ready to hear their diagnosis in stages, and the patient who is satisfied with the diagnosis *tumor* before surgery may some time after ask "What kind of tumor," or "Was it cancer?" The physician must therefore be prepared to give information in doses, in accordance with the patient's current need.

*Case 3.** An example of how a physician may manage and support his patient(s) by assuming a role is illustrated by the following history. Two patients, each aged sixty, one black and one white, were each found to have lung cancer, and were being cared for by the same physician in the same hospital ward. Each of the patients felt himself to be a social outcast, one because he had been an alcoholic and had abandoned his family, and the other because he had been in prison for many years. Because of the similarity in their life situations and the opportunity for their giving each other support and company during their dying processes, the physician encouraged an alliance between the patients, which became notably therapeutic for them. The physician visited the patients daily and participated sometimes in their hilarious bull sessions during which he became a coconspirator and ally with them against their common enemy, the hypocritical society, or the system or the large hospital around them. By his special attention to them in this role he enhanced their self-esteem.

---

*This case is more fully reported in *American Journal of Psychiatry*, *131*:3, March, 1974.

By virtue of his high status and prestige in the medical hierarchy, he was also able to assume the role of omnipotent parent, and to support them directly through the inevitable emotional crises that occurred. In his role as ally or coconspirator, the physician was able to elicit many of the patients' fantasies and fears about what was happening to them and to give them anticipatory guidance, such as when he discussed with them the probable reaction of the survivor after the death of the first patient. Indeed, the surviving patient did become overtly more anxious after his partner died, but was effectively calmed when the physician, in his role as omnipotent parent, told him his time had not yet come. Thus, both patients were maintained in psychological equilibrium until they died by the ability of the physician to personally lend himself to their needs for maintenance of self-esteem and continuing support.

Summary

Our notions of management of the emotional reactions to cancer are based on the physician's and other staff members' becoming alert to the behaviors of these patients so that the behaviors and the total emotional reactions are accorded the values that are needed for careful investigation and necessary intervention. To be sure, we do not negate the humanities in our interest; rather, we are interested in the humanism becoming operational. This can and does occur when the staff is taught and learns to obtain a data base and attends to the data of behavior in a careful manner. Should a patient be told of the diagnosis? The question that *really* frames the answer is, What do the data reveal? Does the patient need nurturing or firmness? The solution will come from what we have observed. Should the spouse or child be used as a therapeutic ally? What does your interview with her or him reveal? Can each physician and staff person perform this task? Certainly each staff person can make valuable cognitive observations. Empathy requires a capacity for vicarious introspection that is variable and, thus, some physicians have limits in this area just as some psychiatrists can do behavioral modification and not be able to do intensive psychotherapy. Therefore, a patient requiring an exploration with attention to inner feelings needs a particular caregiver.

It is clear to us that our primary physician and nurses will continue to do the work of being with our cancer patients and living with their psychological trauma and pain. It is our wish to be of assistance in their understandable state of chagrin and uneasiness by elaborating a scheme of emotional caregiving by focusing on a reasonable approach of observation through collating, diagnosis and finally therapeutic responsiveness. However, we must be mindful of the tasks we have outlined and especially mindful of the support these schema require in the way of assistance from other departments in a hospital, especially the psychiatry division and the cadre of social workers and psychologists required for teaching and supervision.

Suggested Readings

Bowers, M., Jackson, E., Knight, J., et al.: *Counseling the Dying.* New York, Thomas Nelson and Sons, 1964.

Eissler, K.: *The Psychiatrist and the Dying Patient.* New York, International Universities Press, 1955.

Freud, S.: The ego and the id. In *Complete Psychological Works, Standard Edition, Vol. 19,* translated and edited by J. Strachey. London, Hogarth Press, 1961, pp. 13-59.

Kohut, H.: Forms and transformations of narcissism. *Journal of American Psychoanalytic Association, 14*:243-272, 1966.

Kübler-Ross, E.: *On Death and Dying.* New York, Macmillan Co., 1969.

Muslin, H., Levine, S.P., and Levine, H.: Partners in dying. *American Journal of Psychiatry, 131*:3, 1974.

Schoenberg, B., Carr, A.C., Peretz, D., and Kutscher, A.H., (Eds.): *Psychosocial Aspects of Terminal Care.* New York, Columbia University Press, 1972.

Strauss, A., and Glaser, B.: *Anguish: A Case History of a Dying Trajectory.* Mill Valley, California, Sociology Press, 1970.

Weisman, A.: *On Dying and Denying.* New York, Behavioral Publications, 1972.

White, L.P. (Ed.): Care of patients with fatal illness: A symposium. *Annals of New York Academy of Science, 164*:635-896, 1969.

Chapter 6

THE ROLE OF GROUP PROCESS IN STAFF SURVIVAL WITH THE DYING PATIENT

Mahlon S. Hale and John D. Jefferies

THE emotional life of nursing and medical staffs on acute medical and surgical units is inextricably bound up with the levels of severe illness present on these services. This is measured not just by the ratio of survivors and death experienced on such units, but through the intensity of staff relationships with individual patients who seem to represent the keys to staff well-being. How certain patients and their courses of illness become the barometers of staff well-being remains unclear. Patients with hopeless prognoses seem just as likely to be selected as patients whose courses reflect routine recovery and successful treatment.

This report concerns itself with such a dying patient, whose prolonged downhill course was complicated by multiple medical, personal, and social problems. Not the least of these was the impact of her repeated admissions on the morale and group dynamics of the surgery service to which she was frequently admitted. As a liaison psychiatrist (M.H.), one of us witnessed the emergence of staff frustration, disorganization, and depression on this service as repeated admissions failed to reverse this patient's decline.

Subsequently, as an attending physician to this patient on her last two admissions, the psychiatrist unknowingly participated in a group process that resulted in the lessening of staff tensions and facilitated the alleviation of the patient's last major complaint of pain. In retrospect, this final effort was socially restitutive in character; it emerged out of the chaos of the failure of the larger staff group, yet helped to resolve issues that had totally disrupted that group. At the same time, it was able to address the individual patient care issues that were ever present.

Such restitutive psychological maneuvers on a group basis are probably executed frequently on medical and surgical services without staff awareness. In this case, the cast of characters was apparent to the entire service. The multiple purposes of our efforts were not so obvious, however, and psychiatric presence was no guarantee of immediate insight into the nature of these tasks. Such an admission touches upon the intensity of our involvement with our patient for, retrospectively, the reasons for the development of this group process and the nature of the process itself seem clearer to us. In retrospect, we question whether we could not have been more effective had we addressed in totality the issues that are now apparent. Put another way, might we by prospective explication and clarification of group issues deal head-on with the erosiveness that certain events and patients have upon group cohesion?

> Clinical History. This patient was referred to the University of Connecticut Urology Department in May, 1977. In 1954, at the age of thirty-four, she had a carcinoma of the cervix diagnosed and treated by radiotherapy. She was also diagnosed as having adult-onset diabetes, but shortly required insulin. She was also found to have a hiatus hernia, possible angina, hypertension, and intermittent claudication.
>
> The patient worked as a licensed practice nurse in a local hospital and was well known to all the local physicians. During the years between 1954 and 1974, she saw all the general practitioners, internists, cardiologists, and urologists in her immediate area. Most found her a difficult patient to treat because of her aggressive manipulative personality, her refusal to consistently follow treatment orders, and her tendency to change doctors.
>
> In 1970, the patient stopped work as an LPN because "I wasn't up to it." From that time onward, she fought a continuous battle with the state disability department, claiming that she had ceased work for medical reasons. Her demands that she be considered totally disabled led to the alienation of most of the doctors in the community. Eventually, during a disability examination, a Papanicolaou smear was taken. It was found to be positive, and she was referred back to her gynecologist, who confirmed the presence of recurrent carcinoma of the cervix and who performed a hysterectomy in 1974. Following the hysterectomy, her urologic symptoms exacerbated, and she complained continuously of dysuria and frequency.
>
> In April, 1977, she was found to have transitional cell carcinoma of the bladder and was referred to the University because her urologist and the local medical community felt that she was too difficult a patient to treat in the local institutions. She was seen in May of 1977 by the Urology Department, and she was found to have a Grade IV transitional cell carcinoma of the bladder infiltrating the muscle. It was thought that this probably was a consequence of her radiotherapy for the carcinoma of the cervix in 1954. The patient refused a cystectomy and conduit because of her experience in treating patients with ostomies while she was an LPN.

The admission for this diagnosis and the subsequent treatment with external radiotherapy to the bladder, a total dose of 6,400 R, caused a major reaction. The patient had been moderately depressed when seen originally. Following the diagnosis, she became severely depressed. Response to treatment was moderately satisfactory, but she continued to have depression, needing both the hospital psychiatrist and a local psychiatrist during the remainder of her life.

Due to the diagnosis of carcinoma, the State decided to remove the foster child who had been living with her since the age of two (the child was now nine). This caused a major emotional reaction and contributed to her depression. She also complained of rapid deterioration of her eyesight and, during her course of radiotherapy, went to a local ophthalmologist, who performed a cataract extraction, the patient having concealed the fact that she was just concluding a course of radiotherapy.

Between May of 1977 and her death in February of 1980, the patient had fifteen further admissions to hospital. The early admissions were for check cystoscopies, as the patient refused to have cystoscopies without general anesthesia. The cystoscopies showed that the patient's bladder carcinoma was controlled but not eradicated.

This illness in the patient caused a major family reaction. The husband had increasing periods of time off work due to backache and, finally, he had to retire. The youngest son became unemployed for long periods and tended to stay at home. The patient arranged for sale of her house. There was considerable tension generated over the disposal of the monies. One of the sons wished the mother to use the money for a deposit for a house for him; the patient herself wished her husband to have the money. Whenever one of these family problems became acute, the patient was hospitalized for an increase of frequency and pain and failure to respond to analgesics.

Initially, this patient was treated with Tylenol® and codeine, but this totally failed to control the pain. She was found to be allergic to methadone, which gave her hallucinations. In November of 1977, Brompton's Mixture® was started. This was used progressively more frequently and in larger amounts as time went on. It was only, however, used regularly and consistently during the last nine months of her life.

Nine months before death, the patient developed bilateral ureteric obstruction, with elevation of the BUN to 45 and the creatinine to 1.5. Bilateral nephrostomies were inserted. No specific treatment was given for this. The patient began repeatedly diagnosing herself as having a respiratory tract infection and would frequently take long courses of antibiotics, as a result of which she had Candida infections of the mouth and perineum repeatedly. These were controlled by discontinuing the antibiotics and using oral nystatin.

The patient was extremely aggressive in demanding curative treatments whenever there was a relapse of her disease. Quite unconsciously, she would attempt to manipulate doctor against doctor, doctor against nurse, and nurse against nurse. Her depression waxed and waned. She alienated her children, her husband spent all his time catering to her and, in fact, became the stabilizing factor in the family. The unmarried son at home fluctuated between ignoring her condition, arguing with her, and being overly attentive. The patient regarded her stays in hospitals as a break from the emotional tension of her home; but, when she was in hospital, she ended up by inducing the same type of emotional tension that was present in her home among the nursing staff and physicians. In this case, the massiveness of the family's disruption and our patient's characterological style complicated defensive management severalfold.

In spite of the nephrostomy drainage, the patient's pain increased. During her final two admissions, she was attended upon by psychiatrist and urologist together. The Brompton's Mixture in dosages that now controlled the pain left her confused and sedated, much to the increased concern of staff. We elected to substitute levorphanol (Levo-Dromoran®) and dextroamphetamine (Dexedrine®), and we obtained a satisfactory analgesia and increased alertness. The patient began to discuss actively her condition with her physicians and her husband, and she expressed concern that her hospitalizations seemed endless. She decided, in agreement with her husband, that the nephrostomy tubes were prolonging her life unnecessarily and asked for them to be clamped off. This was done. She left the hospital under her husband's care and died at home eight days later. Throughout this period, we and our nurse maintained contact with the patient and her husband. They remained content with their decision, and the husband commented that the turning issue had been the relief of the pain.

Separate from the social disarray of this patient and her family, the medical complications as we describe represent a disheartening prognosis. The azotemic and infectious consequences of urinary obstruction overtly signal failure to patients and physicians alike. Downhill courses become fraught with physical and mental erosion of both patients and their families. The confidence of the caregivers also erodes as they fail to meet either the threat of such illnesses or their complications. The intensification of pain in patients heightens the perception of patient and family members that caregivers are not omniscient and are not competent to handle all situations as patient or family had so inferred when the caregivers used powerful antibiotics to master infection. Parallel perceptions with psychological overtones build in nursing and medical staffs for reasons that have little to do with the battle against hopelessly advanced disease and more to do with symptomatic treatments for the patients and intermittent psychological rescue for the patients' families.

For the liaison psychiatrist, these are familiar issues on hospital

services that specialize in taking care of patients with end-stage illnesses. As a matter of routine, we are involved in the support and protection of permanent staffs against repeated exposure to patients for whom the hope of recovery is negligible and the manifest expectation of gratification for staffs remote.

This is conveniently accomplished by scheduled meetings and rounds maintained with an ambivalent fervor that occasionally approaches religious intensity. Groups form, work, and dissolve as ward issues that remain within familiar expectations arise and ebb. Open agendas are dealt with expeditiously by the group, which relies on collective and individual experience from previous ward experiences and patients. More latent agendas involving relationships with physicians and ward politics are often tolerated by the group for weeks or months before they meet acknowledgment and resolution. In short, patients and issues that fall within the familiar experience of the group are worked with at fairly consistent levels. Even long-term issues that occasionally rise to the surface and affect group members are tolerated, for the lesion is not so painful that it cannot be withstood.

With some patients, however, the group reaction is quite different. Open and latent issues merge and conflictually overpower the group. The perception of ineffectiveness is immediate; the lesion remains open and is constantly painful. Familiar coping styles are found inadequate for the tasks of understanding and working through conflicts. Perhaps what is most painful about such patients is that in some way they remind us that we are not in control of another's destiny. If we were, we surely would not pursue the same issues so constantly with such limited capability for mastery.

This patient's illness and eventual death stimulated more than the usual strivings on the part of the initial support group as it struggled with her multiple admissions. Her presence also released the feelings and maneuverings alluded to among our staff. Her agony and discomfort at times seemed part of her disease and beyond medical control. At other times, her symptoms seemed characterological and refractory to psychological intervention. In the latter part of the past year, the patient's illness took on a terminal haze. Admissions were numerous, brief, and only temporarily effective. General knowledge of her refractory problems created a premonitory ripple effect among nurses, house staff, and attending physicians. When chronic pain was added to her problem list, foreboding and helplessness were added to the problem list carried by the staff.

The apprehension this patient's presence evoked was manifested in other ways. The outpatient nurse found herself in daily contact with the patient and her husband at home. The urologist and psychiatrist would pass in the hall and, from a nod, the psychiatrist would know that the patient was scheduled for admission. Twice in the last months of the patient's life, ward secretaries called the psychiatrist or a staff member of his to advise of an impending admission, without consulting the house staff or the urologist. Members of the nursing staff became indecisive on questions of routine care. Pain medication orders were questioned and delayed. The consequences of these changes were that the psychiatrist no longer consulted, but attended. The urologist no longer attended, but attended constantly. Staff perceptions began to give us not just separate status, but separate responsibility for a patient perceived by staff as beyond control.

Those familiar with theories of group process may recognize the emergence of group process themes developed by the British psychiatrist, Wilfred Bion. Neither the urologist nor the psychiatrist overtly recognized that they were rebuilding a small, workable group unit out of the remnants of a larger, ineffective group that had lost the ability to mobilize its energies to deal with the intractable course of our patient. Yet, we had replicated the course and the experience of the group process that Bion described as functioning on two levels: the *work group* that assigns itself to the primary task of resolving problems in the here and now and, a series of contemporaneous shadow forces, or *basic assumptions* that influence the efforts, none of which may be completely fulfilled (Bion, 1961). These are the basic assumptions of dependency, the basic assumption that the group has coalesced to fight or flight, and the basic assumption of pairing. The assumption of dependency vests its energies in the collective wish to be taken care of by a single leader. The assumption of fight or flight rests on the belief that the group has been created solely to preserve itself and that this may be accomplished either by combat or the very opposite of running away and avoidance. The last basic assumption rests on the wish that the merger or union of individuals will result in collective productivity and salvation.

In more conventional psychiatric settings, we might characterize these basic assumptions as regressive. But, it would seem that within the setting where we found these assumptions in the ascendent, i.e. a surgical unit that frequently experienced multiple difficult admissions, the basic assumptions were neither good nor bad. These assumptions, after all, reflect the internal psychic world where compensatory mechanisms attempt to shore up the bad news that reality is often tougher than we wish to perceive, that under some circumstances hard work will not get the job done, and that any work group will lose its cohesiveness in the face of the threatening perception that it lacks the skills to master the task it believes manifest.

The apprehension and anxiety that undermined the basic work group did give birth to a second group process: a work group comprising the two physicians, the outpatient nurse, the patient, and her husband. With this shrinkage in numbers came a downward revision in expectations and, paradoxically, an increased capability.

The creation of this second work group may be understood by applying Bion's conceptualizations to the initial group. This group was composed of the entire nursing and medical staffs. The urologist was their leader, the psychiatrist an observer. Our outpatient nurse was outside the group, as was the patient, although her preservation was the ostensible work at hand.

Intertwined with the caregiving function of the initial work group lurked the basic assumption of dependency, the belief that if one did a good job, one's own needs would be taken care of. However, as the patient herself moved from crisis to crisis, the basic assumption of dependency began to erode. With that erosion, the group retreated to the basic assumption of fight or flight. However, fighting rapidly proved unsuccessful due to the limitations upon therapeutic stratagems and procedures. Flight, on the other hand, was an acceptable alternative in a medical system with high expectations and other patient responsibilities. The multiple other tasks that the caregivers performed for other patients offered only temporary escape, but could not preserve cohesive behavior towards this particular patient.

Perhaps at the time my colleague and I nodded in the hall, we began to experience the force of the initial work group's marshalling its final basic assumption that focused on the pairing of our presumed skills. This pairing did bring forth what we labeled an alternative strategy. In hindsight, this proved not a concept, but the second working group, whose members merged their primary task and the basic assumptions into a set of mutually acceptable expectations. Inclusion of the patient and her husband substantively changed the group. Previously, she had been the subject but not a member of group efforts, though we do not doubt that some of her residual expectations concerning survival were shared by the group and contributed to the impasse upon which it had floundered.

The task of the second work group was explicit. We would engage in whatever efforts were necessary in order to relieve pain. We would engage in appropriate medical measures to treat sepsis, but we would not be heroic. One of us, our nurse, would maintain continuous monitoring of the patient when she was not in the hospital. The patient herself became specific. She recognized that she was going to die. The pain was what was intolerable; that was what she wished treated.

With the formation of this second work group, we also experienced the positive incorporation of those basic assumptions that compromised the earlier group. First, it became a totally acceptable wish of one member of the group to be taken care of. With explicit guidelines around the issue of analgesia, the group was able to fend off the dependency basic assumption. Caregiving was to be performed in a way congruent with overt expectations. Secondly, we recognized that we had exhausted ourselves over fight and flight issues. The disease and its complications were far advanced. We could neither fight along the lines of cure nor could we flee the outcome of metastatic illness. To acknowledge this dilemma was to make the core issue of the fight and flight basic assumption manifest. In doing this, we became able to deal with the only anticipated outcome, death, in a more rational manner.

From the developmental point of view, the last basic assumption of pairing is also the most advanced and adult-like. Rather than dealing with this assumption as a dissonant element in our alternative strategy, we should like to believe that we successfully integrated a potentially conflictive assumption into the work group by verbalizing a core belief, i.e. that we could, at any cost, attain mastery over pain through effective analgesia. Once we tacitly acknowledged that we could not master the illness, we elected to master the most threatening symptom identified by our patient-member of the group.

Levorphanol was one further step on a logical tree after other analgesics, proven in other situations, had been found ineffective. About the use of the stimulant, we have more questions. The issue of such medications was addressed in the *New England Journal of Medicine* (Forrest et al., 1977), but that study deals with the diminished requirement for morphine when dextroamphetamine is also prescribed. We were reaching not for a reduction in analgesic requirement, but toward a means of remaining in touch with our patient. Although this kind of observation is anecdotal, we believe that the dextroamphetamine kept our patient alert and facilitated her participation in the decision to pursue no more treatment.

Measurement of the effects of this process upon the ward staff also remains anecdotal. What changed for the staff initially was the state of tension by our removal of the symptom. However, even as decisions were being made regarding terminal care, we perceived that the staff still viewed the patient in largely negativistic terms. Herein lies our concern regarding open clarification of the group issues. We were not simply put in the position of taking over the case; that is far too simplistic a view of the group process. If we accept that, then we may be led down a path of incorrect inferences about staff competence. The reality was that our staff was, and is, quite competent. The issue was that efforts became superhuman and increasingly ineffectual, as expectations were not met and basic assumptions began to control the efforts of an increasingly frustrated group. We are not certain that open interpretation of basic assumptions will either be tolerated or used by our major group. On the other hand, our retrospective review has clarified the meaning of our efforts and made comprehensible our motivation for the alternative strategy. We have now started this process of education. Time and experience will tell how this affects our staff well-being and the well-being of our patients.

References

Bion, W.R.: *Experiences in Groups*. London, Tavistock Press, 1961.
Forrest, W.H., Brown, B.W., et al.: Dextroamphetamine with morphine for the treatment of post-operative pain. *New England Journal of Medicine, 296*:712-715, 1977.

Chapter 7

THE FUNCTIONING OF AN ETHICS COMMITTEE IN A COMMUNITY HOSPITAL

WILLIAM F. FINN

EVERY hospital, governmental, voluntary, or proprietary, should have an ethics committee. A community hospital that serves a certain geographical area has a special need for such a committee. The medical staff bylaws provide for all the traditional committees: credentials, medical care appraisal, and infections. The last decade, with the resurgence of biomedical ethics, patient's rights, and preservation of biological life by sophisticated new technological instruments, has created a necessity for health professionals to think about how to treat the human being as well as the patient. Since this subject was not in any curriculum until recent years, there is also a need for such a committee to provide an educational forum.

There are different types of ethics committees, and they have been called by many names: critical care committees, death committees, prognosis committees, optimum care committees, or ad hoc committees. The first name is not comprehensive enough, while the choice of the second one is unfortunate. Perhaps the best known committee is the Critical Care Committee at the Massachusetts General Hospital (Critical Care Committee, 1976). It has a subcommittee called the Optimum Care Committee, which reviews the treatment of the hopelessly ill patient and the utilization of critical care facilities. It was established in 1975 with a psychiatrist as chairman. The other members are a lawyer, an assistant nursing director in charge of intensive care nursing, a medical oncologist, a general surgeon and a lay woman who is a former cancer patient. The committee's function is advisory; the attending physician must request the committee's consultation. When invited, the committee classifies the patient into one of four groups:

1. Maximum therapeutic effort without review
2. Maximum therapeutic effort with daily review
3. Selective limitation of therapeutic effort

4. Discontinuance of therapy

The attending physician may accept or reject the recommendations. Serious differences of opinion lead the director of the Intensive Care Unit (I.C.U.) to request consultation with the chief of service for resolution.

This committee is designed for a limited purpose: classification of seriously ill patients for therapeutic purposes, i.e. triage. It is advisory and does not interfere with the patient-physician relationship. Yet this is a defect since neither the patient when unconscious nor the grieving relatives know that such consultation has been obtained. The composition of the committee is well balanced and includes a lawyer and a former patient.

Activated in 1977, the Montefiore Hospital Committee (Esqueda, 1978) is much more comprehensive since it considers hospital-wide questions of an ethical or a legal nature and provides a forum for such concerns. Also, it acts as an advisory committee on hospital policy to the director. The hospital personnel are represented in a comprehensive and democratic fashion: internists, surgeons, pediatricians, an oncologist, a neurologist, and a resident. This committee is exemplary because it includes a philosopher, a lawyer, an administrator, a social worker, and a patient representative. So far, it has considered patient consent and refusal of treatment and similar issues. Although this committee would not triage dying patients, it would discuss the ethical problems and principles involved. It deserves credit for its comprehensive selection of personnel and for its involvement in all areas of the hospital.

A third type of committee was founded at the hospital of the Albert Einstein College of Medicine in 1975 (Esqueda). It has representatives from many medical specialties as well as administration, nursing, social work, and rehabilitation. The associate dean for medical affairs, the medical director, the chief of nursing, and the chief of administration also attend the monthly meetings held to discuss medical problems with bioethical implications. The intent is to sensitize the hospital personnel to these difficult topics and not to make censurious judgments.

A fourth type of committee is the Quinlan Committee (Levine, 1977; Veatch, 1977), which was established at the Morris View Nursing Home in 1976 in response to the legal decision of Chief Justice Hughes of New Jersey. This committee is based on the 1975 suggestion of Karen Teel and is composed of a chairman who represents the Welfare Board, an attorney, two clergymen, a social worker, and a physician. Its purpose is to assist the family with ethical problems concerning the patient's care or treatment. The court assigned this committee one function in regard to Karen Ann Quinlan, to confirm that "no reasonable possibility of Karen's ever emerging from her present comatose condition to a cognitive, sapient state" existed. So while the committee disclaims this vigorously, it is really a prognosis committee as Veatch points out (1977). It need not be consulted regarding a treatment-stopping decision. The composition of the group is not appropriate to its purpose; it should be composed of physicians, especially neurologists. Although the Quinlan Committee has been basically nonoperative, it has continued as a standing committee at the nursing home.

Veatch, after questioning whether hospital ethics committees function to review medical facts or the ethical and value issues involved in medical diagnosis and treatment, concludes in favor of the latter. He lists four possible tasks for such committees:

1. Review of ethical and other values in individual care decisions
2. Formulation of larger ethical and policy decisions
3. Counseling
4. Prognosis

The above outline of the functioning of four diverse hospital committees shows how each has individualized its committee to conform to its needs and environment.

Hospital medical ethics committees should have three goals:

1. Heightening the level of concern of health professionals who care for dying patients and their bereaved relatives
2. Increasing humane care for dying patients and their grieving relatives
3. Serving as support systems for health professionals who care for critically ill patients

Another committee exists at North Shore University Hospital—a 600-bed facility located in Manhasset, New York, about 17 miles east of New York City on the North Shore of Long Island. With New York Hospital and the Memorial Hospital for Cancer and Allied Diseases, it constitutes a teaching hospital for Cornell University Medical College.

In 1973, a psychiatrist, two social workers, a clinical nurse practitioner, and a gynecologist who were distressed by the routine, perfunctory, apathetic care and/or lack of care for terminally ill patients at North Shore University Hospital discussed how it could be improved. The group pledged allegiance to the three goals noted above and decided that the purpose of an ethics committee would be educational, advisory, and directed toward formulation of hospital policy. It would be a multidisciplinary committee with broad based hospital representation that would concentrate on the most concerned personnel and critical areas of the hospital.

The steering committee consists of a trustee; a lawyer; a community resident; a volunteer; a social worker; and four physicians, a psychiatrist, two internists, and a gynecologist. Membership is open to anyone who works in the hospital or lives in the community, and it includes house officers, medical records personnel, the morgue attendant, community residents, clergy, dialysis attendants, laboratory technicians, and home care personnel. The areas under constant survey are the following:

Emergency Room
Surgical Intensive Care Unit
Medical Intensive Care Unit
Coronary Intensive Care Unit
Delivery Floor
Newborn Nursery
Psychiatry
Oncology Wards
Dialysis Units
Radiotherapy Area

Less critical areas are reviewed as problems arise.

When founded in 1973, this committee was called the Committee on Dying, Death and Bereavement. Its functions have been educational. Monthly meetings consist of case reports of critically ill patients, e.g. Tay-Sachs Disease, brain death; panel discussions of a topic, e.g. "Should cardiopulmonary resuscitation be done on every patient?"; guest lectures; and problem presentations. Judgments are not passed, and anonymity of the source is preserved, if desired.

Suggested changes in policy are sent to the administrator. One of the improvements brought about by the committee is the establishment of private areas in which to speak to relatives and to record hospital autopsy permits. Intense efforts are made to obtain kidney and corneal donations; an outpatient hospice program has been founded; and work toward an inpatient hospice has started. There are liaison psychiatry support systems for professionals, which have become more necessary in an age which attempts to cure without caring.

In 1978, the committee decided that it had attained many of its objectives and that the Dying, Death and Bereavement Committee should be assigned a more appropriate classification related to biomedical ethics. The medical board gave permission for the committee to assume this wider scope, and it was renamed the Committee for Medicine, Society and Ethics. The committee has formed an association with the Department of Philosophy at C.W. Post Center to serve the needs of the community, the university, and the hospital.

An ethics committee should be more than a "death" committee. It should consider all ethical interactions between medicine and the human beings who compose a society.

References

Critical Care Committee: Massachusetts General Hospital Report. *New England Journal of Medicine, 295*:364, 1976.
Esqueda, K.: Hospital ethics committees. *Hospital Medical Staff,* 7:26, 1978.
Levine, C.: Hospital ethics committees: A guarded prognosis. *Hastings Center Report,* 7:25, 1977.
Teel, K.: *Baylor Law Review,* 27:6, 1975.
Veatch, R.: Hospital ethics committees: Is there a role? *Hastings Center Report,* 7:22, 1977.

II.
SPECIFIC PROBLEMS IN UROLOGIC CAREGIVING

Chapter 8

SELF-IDENTIFIED FEARS AND CONCERNS OF BLADDER CANCER PATIENTS

GEORGE SAENZ AND JACQUELYN EDWARDS

Literature

SINCE the 1950s there has been a growing interest in the psychosocial aspects of neoplastic diseases and their possible correlation with emotions. The literature has, however, dealt sparsely with the emotional aspects of bladder cancer. Examples in the literature about emotional problems of bladder cancer patients are for the most part personal accounts having little or no statistical basis. Miller (1977) related the following from "the impressions of personnel who work with these problems":

1. Patients adjust better when they return quickly to their pretreatment life-style.
2. Close supportive contact with the treatment team enhances the patient's ability to adjust to sexual changes resulting from treatment.
3. Patients with bladder cancer are subject to discrimination in the business community.
4. Positive family support is very important in postoperative adjustments.
5. The postoperative life situation must be taken into account when trying to assess the patient's postoperative course.

These conditions appear to be valid from an intuitive standpoint. Having worked with bladder cancer patients for a combined total of thirteen years, we have reached many of the same conclusions. Therefore, it seemed logical to (1) have the bladder patients self-identify their problems and (2) to try to establish whether these self-identified problems remain consistent longitudinally throughout treatment.

Patients and Methods

The study consisted of twenty evaluable bladder cancer patients and two patients not evaluable because they were illiterate. The patients were divided into three groups with reference to amount of disease: (1) Stage O/A, (2) Stage B1, B2, and C, and (3) Stage D1 and D2. The population studied corresponds roughly to the percentage breakdown of cancer of the bladder patients referred to M.D. Anderson Hospital.

The population was comprised of inpatients with cancer of the bladder treated at M.D. Anderson Hospital during February and March, 1980, who agreed to participate. The patient population was made up of four women and sixteen men.

Demographic

The demography of this study from a percentage point of view reflects closely the demography of the bladder population referred to M.D. Anderson Hospital during the years 1969 to 1977.

TABLE 8-I

AGE

	30-35	46-50	51-55	55-60	61-65	66-70	71-75
O/A	1			1			
B/C		1		3	2	3	1
D		1	1	1	1	3	1

TABLE 8-II

RACE

	Black	White
O/A	0	2
B/C	0	10
D	0	8

TABLE 8-III

SEX

Stage of Disease	Male	Female
O/A	2	0
B/C	8	2
D	6	2

TABLE 8-IV

Means of the Questions in Each Category

Category I — Death
Category II — Interpersonal areas of concern to include family, psychogenic, social, and business
Category III — Medically related fears
Category IV — Sex
Category V — Concern for the future
Category VI — Concern about what happens after death

CATEGORY OF QUESTION

Stage of Disease	I	II	III	IV	V	VI
O/A	2.5	2.3	2.4	3.0	3.3	2.3
B/C	2.3	2.4	2.5	1.9	2.8	2.1
D	2.2	2.3	2.3	1.2	2.6	1.6

Construction of the Self-Report Measurement

The self-report instrument was constructed by the authors from interviews of ten inpatients.

The interviews were conducted in the following fashion. All interviews were conducted with hospital inpatients; both authors were present for each interview. Leadership of the interviews was rotated between the two authors.

The patients were informed of the purpose of the study and consented to participate. They were then asked to identify the concerns and worries they or someone in their situation might have experienced in the past month. From these patterned interviews the following categories representing major areas of concern were abstracted: (1) death and mortality fears, consisting of five items; (2) interpersonal areas of concern — to include family, psychogenic, social and business — consisting of twelve items; (3) medically related fears, consisting of eleven items; (4) sexual fears, consisting of three items; (5) concern for the future, consisting of seven items; and (6) thoughts about what happens after death, consisting of two items. A total of forty items were elicited from the preliminary interviews and became the basis of the study. The questionnaire was constructed in such a manner that the different categories were interspersed throughout. One section of eight items, taken from all categories, pertained only to those patients who had undergone a cystectomy. Statistical validation studies were not done on the questionnaire due to limited time.

Administration of Questionnaire to Participants

The twenty participants in the group study were instructed to measure their response to each item by using a five-point scale, ranging from one (1) (never) to five (5) (almost always). The format of the items is a statement beginning with the words, "I worry about....," e.g. I worry about the price of gasoline. The answer choices are (1) never, (2) seldom, (3) frequently, (4) usually, and (5) almost always.

The instructions were to circle the number most appropriate to them. They were basically to respond with their first impression and not to discuss their answers with anyone. From these answers the means of each category were figured.

Results

The results in Category I, Death and Mortality, were essentially the same for all groups, the population mean being around the 2.3 level. The highest incidence of worry occurs in the O/A group at $\bar{x}$ 2.5, the least in the D group $\bar{x}$ 2.2. The B/C group had a $\bar{x}$ 2.3 These figures indicate that the entire population worried about death and mortality between seldom and frequently.

Category II, Interpersonal Areas of Concern, is also essentially the same for all the groups. The B/C group reports $\bar{x}$ 2.4, while the other groups both report $\bar{x}$ 2.3. Again, the entire population reports to worry about interpersonal areas of concern from seldom and frequently.

Category III, Medically Related Issues, falls between seldom and frequently. The B/C reports the highest level of worry at $\bar{x}$ 2.5, followed by the O/A group with $\bar{x}$ 2.4 and the D group $\bar{x}$ 2.3.

Category IV, Sexual Worries, is the lone category in which there appears to be a possible significance between groups. The O/A group reports frequent fears at $\bar{x}$ 3.0 followed by the B/C group reporting seldom fears $\bar{x}$ 1.9. The D group reports $\bar{x}$ 1.2 just above never. Remember that the D group is in the hospital and undergoing chemotherapy and probably near death and would be expected to have fewer sexual concerns. Two of the eight in this group have since died.

In Category V, Concern for Future, the population reported frequent fears around the $\bar{x}$ 3.0 level. Some variance was manifested between groups. The O/A group is at $\bar{x}$ 3.3, the highest level of fear reported in the entire study. The B/C group followed with a $\bar{x}$ 2.8, and the D group rated their fears at the $\bar{x}$ 2.6 level.

Category VI, What Occurs After Death, shows some variance between groups, but the variance is small and rounds out at the $\bar{x}$ 2.0 level (seldom). The O/A group leads at the $\bar{x}$ 2.3 level, followed by the B/C group at $\bar{x}$ 2.1 level and the D group at the $\bar{x}$ 1.6 level. (See Table 8-IV.)

Conclusions

Death as a single issue does not appear to be of overriding worry to the three groups of patients in relation to the other identified categories of worry. It is interesting that all three groups of patients rate the fear of death itself higher than the fear of what happens after death. The O/A group reports more worries about both death itself and what happens after death than either of the other two groups. The B/C group follows in both issues and the D group reports the least worry on both issues. The D group is physically closer to death and therefore may be moving closer to a resolution of their worries in regard to death or may be overwhelmed by the physical demands of their illnesses.

The area of worry that all three groups rated the highest is the future. An average rating of frequently was given by all three groups. The O/A group has worry about the future the highest (3.3 — frequently) rating of the entire study. The B/C and D groups followed in order. This may reflect a greater range of variables that the future encompasses based on the fact that future-oriented thinking implies continued life. Also, it should be pointed out that three of the seven items in this category dealt with possible recurrence of the disease.

The group of patients in the B/C stage of disease has an interesting pattern of self-identified worries. It should be remembered that this is the group adjusting to a cystectomy. Their greatest areas of worry are the future, interpersonal worries, and medically related worries. In both the interpersonal and medically related categories, the B/C patients reported a higher level of worry than the O/A and the D groups. The higher level of worry in these two areas could reflect the stress of surgery and its adjustments.

As would be intuitively thought, the O/A group is more worried about sex. The B/C group seems to defer worries about sex in order to deal with recurrence, possible surgery, and possible death. The lowest rating of 1.2 in the entire study is given by the D group to the category of sex. Again, conventional wisdom could hypothesize this.

Summary

These findings have some implication in how the social worker and other members of the health care team can help bladder cancer patients deal with the emotional aspects of their illness. Because all three groups rated the category of future worries highest, this study would suggest counseling be done from a future-oriented perspective. It appears that self-identified problems change as the patient progresses through his/her disease.

This study would suggest that beginning patients (O/A) are willing to admit to a higher level of worry in all categories and may be more open to counseling intervention. The D patients report fewer worried in all categories, perhaps reflecting (1) a greater resolution of worries, (2) a greater ability to deny, and (3) a tendency toward isolating themselves. In helping this group of patients deal with death it can be pointed out that death is not the overwhelming worry but is a steady issue throughout the study and across groups. Also, it can be associated with the high level of worry about the future.

Reference

Miller, R.N.: The emotional problems of patients with bladder cancer. *Cancer Research, 37*:2789-2791, 1977.

Chapter 9

CARE OF DYING PATIENTS WITH INCIDENTAL BLADDER OUTLET OBSTRUCTION

HARLAN A. KUTSCHER

THE urologist often is consulted by a male patient's primary physician to help take care of the man's difficulty in voiding. To help this man, the urologist carries the usual armamentarium of diagnostic techniques and methods of urinary diversion. The urologist is accustomed to consultation since this forms the basis of his practice. He may also feel reasonably comfortable dealing with patients he has previously treated who may be dying since he has had a chance to know this person over time. However, a consultation to see a previously unknown man who is dying presents obvious difficulties.

A relevant example is a seventy-six-year-old former newspaper editor with metastatic oat cell carcinoma who developed urinary retention. He had a long history of bladder outlet obstructive symptoms which were treated by his primary physician. When seen initially by the urologist, he was undergoing his first chemotherapy treatment. His primary physician was not optimistic. The patient presently had a Foley catheter in place, but was apparently uncomfortable with the tube because of symptoms secondary to urethritis. The logical choice for a person with a few months to live was to place a suprapubic tube. However, in talking with the patient, it became apparent that he was unhappy with the indwelling catheter, not only because it was physically uncomfortable, but because he was uncomfortable with the idea of living and probably dying with a tube to replace a bodily function. His prostate was palpably greater than 50 grams on rectal examination and probably not amenable to transurethral resection. A long discussion with the patient ensued about the ease of placement and use of suprapubic tube. However, he was very upset by the prospect of the suprapubic tube and asked if there wasn't some way he could avoid having the tube and being able to void on his own for what he estimated were several remaining months of his life.

This question essentially took on the proportions of a dying man's wish. For this reason, the plan was established to perform a cystoscopy and, if possible, to perform a transurethral resection of the prostate. If the prostate was too large for this procedure, however, the patient was prepared to accept placement of a suprapubic tube.

Unfortunately, a preoperative white blood cell count was only 1,100 because of his chemotherapy and his surgical date had to be postponed. But just as importantly, the patient's primary doctor did not feel a major operation was appropriate in a dying patient. The problem became further exacerbated when the patient's indwelling Foley catheter clogged and the patient became even more leery of having any tube. He was readmitted the next week (when his white blood cell count had returned to normal), and he underwent cystoscopy. The prostate was markedly enlarged, almost two loop lengths long, and a transurethral resection was felt to be a major undertaking. Under ordinary circumstances, a gland this size would have been treated with open prostatectomy, but even the patient had agreed that an open operation with its more significant morbidity and recovery time would not be worthwhile. Therefore, a suprapubic tube was inserted, and a new course of chemotherapy was begun.

Interestingly, the outcome of the suprapubic tube insertion was what seemed initially the treatment of choice before talking to the patient, and the suprapubic tube was what the primary physician wanted all along. In this particular situation, the primary physician was the individual not sufficiently attentive and responsive to the patient's needs, looking for a quick solution rather than one that would best suit the patient's emotional as well as medical needs.

Several facets of this situation also deserve further note. First of all, the patient lives alone and is self-sufficient. He is weak, but not debilitated. Many patients in this same situation are too weak to need to be concerned about being independent enough to void. Other patients at least have family members to help care for complications involving catheter care. Of course, family members' opinions about the care they are prepared to give are important in this regard.

Finally, in the event that care may eventually be needed in a nursing home, certain types of patient needs may make placement difficult in certain areas. The size of this patient's prostate made intermittent catheterization impractical because of difficulty getting by the gland. Patients who might be managed by this technique in particular might not be good candidates for nursing home placement, or perhaps in some areas, the additional care would raise the level of reimbursement for the patient and make it easier to place him in a nursing home.

This discussion is not meant to be a comprehensive discussion of all the treatment options available to bladder outlet obstruction in dying patients, but mainly it is designed to serve as an illustration of the potential problems that may arise among a urologist acting as a consultant, a patient, and his primary care physician and the ensuing difficulties that may develop from certain forms of medical treatment. At least the patient has the final say as to whether any operative intervention will take place. However, the patient cannot have an operation, which he would really benefit from, if the consulting urologist does not carry with him a sufficiently open mind to allow for unusual uses of his therapeutic armamentarium.

Chapter 10

BENEMORTASIA

Charles D. Saunders

PHYSICIANS have always made decisions affecting the life and death of patients. The management of patients with advanced cancer can be difficult and often requires the cooperation of several physicians. The urologist becomes involved when tumors outside the urinary tract obstruct the flow of urine from the kidneys to the bladder.

The ureters are the tubes that convey the urine from each kidney to the bladder. Ureteral obstruction is common in patients with advanced pelvic cancers. As the tumors grow (from the bowel, female or male organs), they may surround the ureter, compress it, and finally obstruct the flow of urine through this small tube. When this occurs bilaterally, there can be no urine output, or anuria. Acute life threatening uremia results, and the urologist is called to perform a urinary diversion.

A urinary diversion is an operation to bypass the obstruction. It most commonly consists of surgically exposing a kidney, placing a drainage tube in its inferior pole, and bringing this tube out the patient's side (a nephrostomy). An alternative procedure would be to cut the ureter above the area of obstruction and to sew it directly to the skin (a cutaneous ureterostomy).

As a result of each procedure, the kidney will again function to rid the body of lethal toxins. In both procedures there is a constant leakage of urine from the diversion site on the skin, and an external collection device or bag must be worn. In addition, such a urinary diversion is a major surgical procedure with an associated morbidity and mortality of its own. The urinary diversion prolongs life by relieving the imminent threat of death from renal failure and uremic poisoning, but it has no effect on the primary disease that caused the urinary obstruction in the first place. Requests for diversion are urgent, emotionally charged, and frequently raise ethical and legal questions. Patients with this problem have a limited life span and should not be subjected to operations requiring long periods of hospitalization with possible complications unless truly necessary.

In this setting it is difficult to apply traditional criteria for determining operability since the benefits of an operation in patients with advanced cancer often are ill-defined and the risks are considerable. There is usually tremendous pressure from the patient's physician, oncologist, radiotherapist, or family.

The decision by the urologist to perform a life-prolonging urinary diversion should be the joint responsibility of the patient, his family, and physicians and should be based upon the merit of each individual case. The goal of this therapy should be to prolong a life that is reasonably comfortable, useful, and dignified. The urologist in this setting must be the one who informs, advises, and recommends a course of action for the patient to choose. The patient alone without such advice and information will not understand the consequences and could not, therefore, make an intelligent decision.

There are no universal rules for the urologist to follow as each such patient presents unique circumstances. But some guidelines would be helpful. If the urologist is to truly communicate with the patient and his family, both should be aware of the diagnosis. Otherwise, there can be no true understanding of the options available. Even when well informed, however, a patient who is quite ill, especially with a terminal illness, is often confused, anxious, and unable to clearly grasp the significance of the situation. The patient, therefore, may remain unclear about what he wants for himself. Under these circumstances, he may all the more rely upon the advice of his physicians. It may become even more confusing if the various specialists involved offer different opinions as to the benefits of prolonging life. It is most important, therefore, that the patient's physicians consult with one another and reach a consensus before making recommendations to the patient as individuals.

Patients likely to benefit from diverting procedures in the face of anuria and recurrent cancer are those who are without widespread cancer, well nourished, active, and remain highly motivated even after the possibilities and problems of a diverting procedure have been explained thoroughly (Schoenberg, 1979, p. 315). There is no evidence that the duration of the disease prior to the urinary diversion carries any prognostic value. Those with a longer history of cancer do not derive any greater benefit from the diverting procedure than those patients more recently diagnosed (Holden et al.,

1979, p. 19; Brin, 1975, p. 619). Severe ureteral obstruction is an extremely late stage of the malignant disease.

Life-prolonging urinary diversions must be considered for those patients who have not had a chance to have a satisfactory course of therapy for their primary tumor. Even if treatment methods are still available affording some chance of palliating the symptoms, then urinary diversion should be used to prolong life so that these methods may be tried. Anticancer programs are doomed to failure in the severely uremic patient. Ideally, the disease should still be localized for further therapy to hold the possibility of survival. If the disease is advanced, it should be one with an unpredictable natural history so that a survival time of at least several months could be possible.

When the above criteria are not followed, the post diversion patient frequently exhibits a downhill course with sepsis, pain, weakness and dies weeks or months later without ever leaving the hospital. Such was the course with 43 percent of those patients in Grabstald's series (1973, p. 217). In Holden's series of 218 patients only 50 percent achieved two months of useful life (1979). Brin studied forty-nine patients undergoing urinary diversion; the average survival was 5.3 months with only 50 percent alive at three months, and 22.7 percent alive at six months. Following diversion, 63.8 percent of survival time was spent in the hospital. Twenty patients required a total of twenty-nine additional operative procedures after urinary diversion, which indicates that the urinary diversion itself is not without its own complications. The vast majority of patients had bouts of sepsis, hematuria, nausea, vomiting, abdominal pain, and blood transfusions (1975). However, in Schoenberg's series of six carefully chosen patients, five patients were considered successes insofar as they lived at home and engaged in normal activities (1979).

If all reasonable methods that might affect the primary disease have been tried and failed, then little is to be gained by urinary diversion except to keep the patient alert while he dies of cancer in a short time. Urinary diversion could reverse an inevitable uremic death and substitute a prolonged painful ordeal for the patient and his family. The uremic state itself affords considerable comfort and relief of pain and freedom to die with dignity.

Urinary diversion should not, therefore, usually be performed when the patient is experiencing pain that is no longer responsive to medical management. Diversions should be avoided in situations where adequate trials of all existing therapeutic modalities have been employed and there is no prospect for further therapy after diversion. Emotional or mental deficiency that would preclude adequate management of the urinary diversion (nephrostomy or ureterostomy with associated appliances) is also a contraindication to diversion.

In summary, urinary diversion should be used to prolong life in patients with terminal illnesses only after careful consideration of the patient's medical and emotional status. The urologist should serve as a forceful guide to a family and patient who have been made as fully aware as possible of the situation. The oncologist, radiotherapist, family physician, and urologist must together examine all aspects of the patient's present and future conditions. New medical life support systems can prolong life without dignity or purpose. Urinary diversion is one such modality. Yet, the quality of existence can be as important as the quantity.

A competent person has the right to refuse medical treatment, even if it means death. Many physicians react to the terminally ill patient's refusal of treatment and choice of death as a tragic mistake. They may even order psychiatric consultations in order to change the patient's mind. Some physicians feel that they are not adequately fulfilling their mission to prolong life by allowing such a decision to occur. They feel a sense of failure in not utilizing the knowledge they have worked so hard to attain. Others are concerned about legal reprisals in allowing a patient to die. Recent court decisions, however, have clearly indicated that a competent individual has the right to refuse treatment. No court has overridden a competent person's decision to refuse treatment in any case involving a more invasive procedure than a blood transfusion. A competent person is legally defined as one who is able to understand the consequences of his actions. Therefore, to be medically competent, the patient must be informed about his disease and contemplated procedures.

Physicians must maintain flexibility in dealing with terminally ill patients. They must not become technicians who follow a set course of action no matter what the circumstances. It is not sufficient to be able to employ the latest scientific advances in treating a disease. One must be able to take into account the person who has the disease and plan a course of therapy that will consider all of his or her needs—emotional as well as physical.

Benemortasia connotes a good death resulting from a disease or disability being allowed to take its course or have its effect while providing the patient palliative drug treatment for pain without any therapeutic intent (Young, 1978, p. 304). As stated above, each patient must be individually considered. Urinary diversion as part of a therapeutic plan will definitely benefit some patients. Others, however, should not be denied, no matter how well meaning a physician's motives are to provide therapy, the choice of a relatively comfortable, dignified benemortasia.

References

Brin, E., et al.: Palliative urinary diversion for Pilou malignancy. *Journal of Urology, 113*:619, 1975.

Grabstald, H., and McPhee, M.: Nephrostomy of the cancer patient. *Southern Medical Journal, 66*:217, 1973.

Holden, S., et al.: The rationale of urinary diversion in cancer patients. *Journal of Urology, 121*:19, 1979.

Schoenberg, H.W., et al.: Urinary diversion for ureteral obstruction in the presence of recurrent colon carcinoma. *Journal of Urology, 122*:315, 1979.

Young, E.: Reflections of life and death. In C. Garfield (Ed.): *Psychosocial Care of the Dying Patient*. New York, McGraw Hill, 1978.

Chapter 11

UROLOGICAL CARE OF THE TERMINAL CANCER PATIENT

Elliot L. Cohen

PRACTICING urologists treat many cancer patients, but certain situations present more acute problems of management. Perhaps the most difficult decision to make is whether to perform urinary diversion on uremic cancer patients. Ureteral obstruction and uremia can occur in those urology patients with prostate and bladder cancer. However, patients with gynecologic or colon malignancies — not urological disorders — can also suffer from uremia.

If we are familiar with the patient, we may have time to anticipate the development of uremia and plan with the patient and the family what measures should be taken in the event of this complication. There are times, though, when a patient comes under our care and there has been no opportunity to develop a rapport with him or the family. In our institution, the presence of an active dialysis unit also complicates the decision-making process. Although dialysis is not undertaken with the sole intention of preserving the life of a terminal cancer patient, there are occasions when a patient is brought to the hospital on an emergency basis and found to be uremic. Dialysis is instituted before all the facts of the case are known. Obviously, this presents a new problem for the urologists: Should we continue the dialysis with the hope of performing a urinary diversion when the patient's condition stabilizes or should we terminate the dialysis and let the patient die?

An eighty-six-year-old man was admitted to the intensive care unit from a nursing home. The patient was severely obtunded and was found to be uremic, but the details of his history were not clear on admission. Family members were contacted, and it became apparent that although they had not been in close touch with the patient in recent years, they wanted everything possible done for him.

Dialysis was instituted; the patient's condition stabilized; and he proved to be a fairly alert and somewhat cantankerous individual. The details of his history revealed that he had been operated on multiple times for bladder cancer and that invasive bladder cancer was probably the cause of his uremia. Since dialysis had already been instituted, the urologist was approached to perform urinary diversion. Consent for the surgery was given by the family, but the patient refused to submit to any operation; he said he had been through enough. After appropriate consultations were obtained to ascertain that the patient was capable of making this decision, the family was told that his wishes would be respected. Finally, the case was presented to the hospital's No Code Committee (*see* below). To avoid any confusion about what to do when the patient again became obtunded from uremia, proper documentation was recorded on the patient's chart. Dialysis was stopped, and the patient died a short time later.

Other difficulties arise in the management of patients with colon cancer, specifically those who have undergone abdominal perineal resection. When ureteral obstruction occurs after this procedure, the cause is almost invariably recurrence of the primary cancer. When uremia and ureteral obstruction occur, along with evidence of widespread metastases, decisions about proper management become somewhat simpler to make. In some cases, however, obstruction occurs despite a completely negative metastatic workup. The possibility then exists that the obstruction may be caused by fibrosis or some other surgical factor, and the management becomes more difficult.

A patient with known metastatic disease was admitted to the hospital. Cystoscopy and biopsy of the bladder revealed evidence of colon cancer invasive to the bladder. All chemotherapy and radiotherapy palliative measures had been exhausted. The patient was experiencing some pain, which was partially relieved by medication. In spite of our initial reluctance, the patient and his family firmly wanted his life preserved. A nephrostomy was performed. Under the continued care of our cancer support group, the patient lived several months, and he and his family were grateful for the additional time they had together. Of course, nephrostomy is not always the answer. In a documented series of 218 nephrostomies, 43 percent of them were done on Friday, Saturday, and Sunday—with 26 percent done on Friday night. It is apparent that other than purely medical factors play a part in the decision to perform urinary diversion. Since major life-threatening complications occurred in 45 percent of this series, the procedure was not without its own risks. Perhaps the most significant statistic is that only 50 percent of the patients with advanced disease achieved two months of useful life.

Recently, urinary diversion has become simpler by the use of internal permanent ureteral catheters such as the Gibbons catheter. Also, percutaneous nephrostomy may be performed, allowing the nephrostomy tube to be inserted without a major operative procedure. However, in view of the above data regarding results of nephrostomy, we should probably use the same criteria for patient selection before employing these simpler methods since we are unlikely to produce any change in the ultimate fate of the patient.

The No Code Committee in our hospital is actually the medical practice board committee. Nurses are required to call a code 66 for an emergency resuscitative team to treat a patient who has had a cardiac or respiratory arrest. No discretion is permitted if the patient is a terminal cancer patient. To avoid the expense and futility of this situation, the patient's own attending physician may call a meeting of the committee, whose members are representatives from anesthesia, cardiology, surgery, neurology, administration, and the clergy. If the committee agrees unanimously that no code should be called, the physician can write a note on the patient's chart indicating that the patient is terminally ill with no hope of recovery or remission and that the patient and/or family request that no resuscitative measures be instituted. If the patient is in a position to give consent, his consent is needed. The note on the chart will be honored by the nursing staff. Each no code patient is reviewed weekly by the committee to determine any change in status.

Chapter 12

A HOSPITAL CANCER SUPPORT GROUP

KATHLEEN A. WEBER

WHEN a few professionals acknowledged their discomfort in being with dying patients, an army chaplain who was doing a rotation at our hospital (United States Public Health Service Hospital, Staten Island, New York) started to meet with the chief of oncology and the radiation oncologist. He told them that our hospital was like many others: "You do a great job of providing medical and surgical care for patients, but when it comes to providing emotional support for patients and families, you fall flat on your face." He brought into the open the problems confronting hospital staff who care for terminally ill patients. We are uncomfortable with dying patients, and we do not know what to say to their families.

An initial group was set up to explore what had been done in other areas regarding interaction with dying patients and their families. The members of the group decided to start a hospital support group. The oncologist selected twenty patients with a life expectancy of one to five years to attend the group. It was felt that by the time the patient reached the terminal stage of illness, a support system would be in place to help him. The group was an open forum where individuals could share their fears and concerns, and it worked well.

The professional committee for the group is composed of doctors, nurses, social workers, a dietary specialist, an occupational therapist, a physical therapist, a health educator, chaplain, public health nurse, and a pharmacist. I serve as coordinator and am the only paid staff member of the group. The other professionals are involved in the group because they want to be, not because they have been assigned to it.

We have expanded to include about 200 families in the cancer support group meetings. Patients and their families meet with us as professionals to learn as much as they can about diagnoses and how to participate in the management of their disease. We have contact with patients from the time of diagnosis instead of only at the terminal stage of illness. We allow the patient and the family to participate and to make decisions regarding their therapy and their death as well as how they live for the remainder of their life.

One thirty-year-old man had been seen both by urology and other departments within the hospital. When I walked into his room one day, he said to me, "Kathy, I can't die in this hospital. Hospitals are inhumane and dehumanizing." I said, "Tom, if your wife can deal with it and we can support you at home, I'll make sure you go home." The visiting nurse, I, and our doctor, who agreed to make house calls, supported this young man and his family at home. Before he died, he said to me, "You know, I really have to thank you and the cancer support program because you eliminated a lot of the bureaucracy of medicine. You are part of our family. If you are able to be here, I want you here when I die." His thanks to us was a request that contributions made in his memory be given to support our program. We have been able to grow because of this.

Our professional committee meets once a week to discuss inpatients and to plan for patient/family education and professional education. As part of professional education, we have guest speakers who have talked about the hospice movement, pain control, and other pertinent topics.

The patient support meetings are not just an emotional support system for patients. The first Thursday of every month is an education session, and the patients determine the agenda. We have covered radiation therapy, chemotherapy, exercise, and sexuality. We have also discussed what laboratory tests mean. The patients have planned and participated in a brunch where patients and their families met with the professionals to share a little social life instead of just considering illness and death.

We have done something unique for a program like ours; the professionals in our program are volunteers. When they found that they were not meeting the needs of the patients in the hospital, the professionals decided to individually support a patient and family. Once a patient comes into the cancer support program and agrees that he would like to participate, he is assigned a professional volunteer who not only shares the expertise of his own field but also becomes a very important listener. One does not have to be a psychologist or a specially trained person to provide loving care and a listening ear.

The reports from our patients and their families have verified that the cancer support professionals have become an extended family to those who need someone to lean on and that we all "get by with a little help from our friends." Our bereavement program follows families for at least one year after the death of their loved one.

Our focus is to care about people. A patient came into my office and asked me, "How can you deal with this program? Every one of your patients dies." I answered, "You know, you are right, and sometimes I get sad and cry when I miss somebody. But I think I have the most beautiful job in the hospital because you give me as I give you." Caring comes through in every discipline in our hospital. I have found dieticians who make better support persons than I do. I have followed them all, and I am what my title calls me, a coordinator. I make sure that the patient does have someone to rely on. I am on call twenty-four hours a day and if I am not there, someone else takes my place. I believe that each hospital should have a system to help patients and families resolve some of their fears. I believe physicians should be team leaders. We cannot have a viable support program without physicians' involvement. However, physicians can utilize a support program such as this to expend their valuable time more profitably by using the team approach and developing other professional liaisons between patients and family members.

Chapter 13

URINARY INCONTINENCE

KATHERINE F. JETER

URINARY incontinence is an inability to control micturition—to control your water. The big issue is that in our culture incontinence is a very shaming situation. Anyone who is incontinent is embarrassed and ashamed until the incontinence is resolved in a satisfactory manner. Of course, what is satisfactory for one person may not be satisfactory for another.

Physicians tell me they have not noticed these effects of incontinence on their patients. I respond that we all have ways of turning off and turning on what patients say. As an enterostomal therapist, I hear more than anyone I know because I have had counseling training to listen and to elicit. I hear what patients know they are not allowed to say elsewhere.

Incontinence has never received much attention in nursing school. The solution, from a nurse's point of view, should not be pads and diapers. *Dry* is the solution, not more absorbency. Remember that, and the patient's whole outlook on living with incontinence will be significantly changed. If you walk into the room and smell urine, something is inadequate about the nursing care.

In 1969, I went to many manufacturers of surgical and medical supplies to present the problems of incontinence. The companies were not interested; they wanted me to define the market. I told them that I did not know or care, that marketing was their problem, and incontinence, mine. Now nearly every one of these companies has a task force on incontinence. Unfortunately, that does not mean they are closer to solutions. The incontinence devices available today (the McGuire Urinal, the Cunningham Clamp) can be found in an early Sears & Roebuck catalog. Today's Cunningham Clamp is plastic and foam instead of metal and sponge, but it's still a Cunningham Clamp.

There is a stigma about urinary or fecal incontinence that goes back to toilet training. In everything we read and everything we are taught, if you can't control your urine or your gas or your stool, you are in a terrible situation. A baby is supposed to be incontinent for only eighteen months. There isn't any culture in the world — Mexican, Vietnamese, African — that has not set a time at which urinary and fecal control is expected. The times may vary from culture to culture, but the time and place are definite. In our culture, it's "I have graduated from diapers and now I can go to school." We go to school at two years of age, yet many schools will not let kids in unless they are continent of urine and stool.

In 1970, when I was at Columbia–Presbyterian Medical Center (New York City), one of the main reasons urinary diversions were performed was to make it possible for incontinent children to go to public school. When parents met together in the clinic, they swapped stories about problems and solutions. Children are mercilessly and horribly embarrassed by their friends. It has not been long since a spanking resulted from incontinence. A boy I met at that time had a very ingenious mother. She clipped the lining of his raincoat, and in his raincoat he pinned the pads that he would need all day. He could go into the bathroom and unpin one of these pads and change there without the embarrassment of carrying a satchel. We had another patient who was a little older. He shaved the hair on his chest and taped pads on his chest and his back so that he could go into restrooms and peel them off.

An eighteen-year-old boy reported that he dropped out of school when a classmate sprayed Lysol® on him from behind when he got up to recite. One of the solutions found at our clinic was that black fabric does not show urine. The place began to look like an Amish colony. I can never forget Sidney, who said that the most exciting thing about his ostomy was that he could put away his black pants and wear khaki and baby blue and all kinds of neat colors.

With adults, we have to consider disposing of about a liter and a half of urine every twenty-four hours. Since cloth is not going to disguise all that water, we have a real management problem with the collection of liquid, the odor, and the clothes. What's a girl to do in a bathing suit?

We had a sixteen-year-old male patient whose scrotum had been nearly eaten through by urine. He was a spina bifida patient, had no feeling, and was beyond the age where it is acceptable for his mother to be examining him (there was no father at home). His medical problem caused alarm, but no one had been alarmed by the fact that he was perfectly miserable. He chose ostomy and was so pleased with it that he ended up recommending it to other people. For him, the procedure was a real salvation, although all my patients may not see it that way. Other problems linger for this young man, including the fact that he never made any friends or that he did not learn how to play with other kids because he was embarrassed.

Middle-aged women also have a problem, and women who have had babies are subject to incontinence. I know about this intimately because it has not been too long since I had my fortieth birthday. Incontinence now is a common subject of conversation. My mother-in-law told me that she stopped entertaining the ladies for luncheon in her home because she has blue damask upholstery on her dining room chairs. When her friends laughed, they piddled on her chairs. One of the recommendations I heartily make to all obstetricians, gynecologists, and ladies who have babies are squeezing exercises begun the first week after childbirth and continued forever.

Incontinence is a problem for sixty percent of all persons over 70 years of age. One sneeze, one cough, one giggle, and that's it.

We should talk to prostatectomy patients before surgery about the possibility of incontinence, and the necessity for doing some squeezing exercises after surgery. Then the patient would not be alarmed with a problem, and he would be actively involved in making the problem as minimal as possible. Many men have problems with incontinence as they get older whether or not they have had a prostatectomy. Some have incontinence and do not want to tell the doctor about it because they are afraid that something was not quite right about the operation. It is so simple to talk ahead of time, to help them get the feel of the exercises so they can start them immediately after the operation.

Then there are the problems about collection devices. At urological meetings the urologists always say, "Yes, we put external devices on our male patients." Which device? "Oh, the team comes around and they handle that." Many condom catheters are appropriate for a virile, twenty-five-year-old male who is still having erections. But if you want to use one on a sixty-five-year-old man after a radical prostatectomy, you might as well try to put toothpaste back in a tube. In some hospitals, they put a rigid penile prosthesis in a flaccid penis to allow for the application of a collection device. Don't be too confident about external collection devices.

If you are looking for a female incontinence device, you have a long way to go. About the best we have is a shower cap with some cellucotton in it. A new adult diaper has been market tested. Nursing homes love this diaper because it holds twice as much as the others, and it doesn't leak. But if you can imagine wearing the same pair of trousers or the same size skirt that you have always worn with this new maxidiaper, you will understand that it has created as many problems as it solves.

The problem among people today is that there is insufficient understanding. The medical and nursing professionals have not made demands on industry. In the Gemini space program, one of the most significant problems was urine collection. They had an elaborate system of molding the penis of each astronaut and making custom-designed urosheaths.

Here we are in the 1980s with nothing better than a maxidiaper. We must specify what we need and what our patients need: They need dryness and something small and convenient (not an extra suitcase or a pad pasted on the chest). We need new male and female incontinence devices that will solve many of the problems and promote human dignity.

Author's note: This chapter was transcribed from a taped lecture.

Chapter 14

URINARY TRACT DISABILITY

Peter N. DeSanctis

ONE of the earliest demands made upon a young child is for excretory continence. It is the focus of parental concern from the earliest time, and with the possible exception of the ability to feed properly, this is the child's most important achievement. If it is delayed, unhappy consequences are assured. One can only speculate on how much grief awaits the child who has delayed urinary control. If the defect should be a permanent one, the child may anticipate an unhappy life in which he or she is certain to be a pariah. Various techniques must be called upon, and these are more or less successful but are invariably kept secret and not to be shared with anybody but the closest and most understanding friends. Yet, permanent disability of this kind is really uncommon. With the exception of an unfortunate few, we have all managed to accomplish this element of physiological maturity. With bladder control, anything is possible; without it, serious social and career limitations exist.

It may be helpful to define normal urinary function and then proceed to the problems of those who are chronically and even acutely ill. Normal bladder function involves these chief features: (1) capacity, (2) sensation, and (3) complete emptying. They interact in subtle ways so that we are hardly aware of them in an undiseased state. In a normal situation, the bladder, unlike any other part of the body, does its job best by hardly doing anything at all. It fills slowly, makes us aware of its distention gradually, and empties quickly. Assuming that the bladder is emptied four to five times a day and that each event might occupy as much as a minute or so of the 1,440 minutes in a day, we can estimate that the bladder uses only a total of five or six minutes to perform its entire daily function correctly. What happens if those brief minutes do not pass as they are meant to?

It is necessary to mention some of the problems encountered in all urologically disabled patients, including those with upper tract disease. Since the entire urinary tract is anatomically and physiologically interrelated, disease that starts in one part may soon affect every other part. This is clearly seen in the neurologically disabled patient whose initial lower urinary tract infection may ultimately end in the complete loss of renal function.

The management of patients with acute urological disease may be undertaken without hospitalization. Indeed, the acute onset of urinary symptoms may occur at any time in the course of a chronic illness. The principles of management of the febrile patient, from whatever cause, are generally well understood and are directed at the source of the fever. If the patient has an uncomplicated urinary tract infection, selected antibiotics, fluids, rest, and local or systemic analgesics may be sufficient. If the patient is very young or very old, special thought must be given to dehydration. Certain infections may predispose to stone formation which adds additional problems over the long term, especially if infections are recurrent and (even worse) if they are persistent.

The point is, however, that patients chronically ill from other organic diseases are even more susceptible to complete disruption of the urinary system. Chronically ill patients, whose health is precariously balanced, develop acute urinary or pulmonary complications that ultimately represent a final onslaught causing death. Most hospitals and health professionals see acute disease routinely and are expert in its management. If there is an area in which we are deficient, it is the delivery of care to the chronically ill or disabled. Chronic upper urinary tract disease may be classified in a number of ways. One category of illness is medical and includes such parenchymal diseases as glomerular nephritis, diabetic nephropathy, pyelonephritis, and nephrosclerosis. There are, however, a large number of patients with chronic renal disease that in other circumstances might be surgically curable; however, surgery is withheld because of technical limitations, the age, and the general condition of the patient. In this group, we might expect patients with advanced cancer, some with single calculi, some who have had unsuccessful previous surgery for obstruction, some with chronic renal disease from tuberculosis, and so forth. Both categories of patients, medical and surgical, may endure for a lengthy period, their care undertaken in a variety of locations (in their own domiciles; in nursing homes, with occasional hospitalizations for specific indications, such as renal dialysis, or for care of an acute exacerbation of pain or fever; or in hospitals).

In general, however, most hospitals are not prepared to care for chronic upper tract disease over the long term, nor should they be required to. If a longer hospitalization is needed, other delivery systems may be required. Although a hospital is suitable for some, a large number of patients with serious illness receive substandard care at home because there is simply no other place for them. The choices then are (1) the patient's home (perhaps with some help from a visiting nurse service), with traumatic results on other members of the household, particularly when only an elderly spouse is available; (2) terminal care facilities, which are extremely costly to the family or society as a whole; and (3) the acute care hospital, which is not prepared to handle a long-term problem.

As we become more expert at prolonging life, we continue to complicate matters. As professionals, we can identify the problem, but the solution has not been in our purview. What we do with our old and disabled is a philosophical issue. As long as we and our families remain healthy, we are safe; however, we should remember that we all become ill. Very few of us pray for a long and lingering demise. Unfortunately, we have become so skillful at saving lives that this often happens.

The ideal management of patients with chronically diseased lower urinary tracts depends upon four considerations: (1) the problem itself with all of its manifestations and symptoms, (2) the reason for the problem, (3) the age and sex of the patients, and (4) the resources available. What is correct for an elderly male dying of prostatic carcinoma may not be relevant to a young woman disabled by multiple sclerosis.

We can easily identify a number of symptoms encountered by the patient—pain, infection, bleeding, and voiding dysfunction. Chronic pain demoralizes at any age, but the very young and very old are most susceptible. In many attempts to forestall narcotic addiction, we allow patients to suffer unnecessarily by withholding proper analgesics in correct doses. This might be a realistic fear, but we must not be overly restrictive in the use of medication. One of the most terrifying aspects of chronic disease, including terminal disease of any kind, is the suffering that may accompany it. We have the means to intercept it, and we should utilize any and all techniques available with scientific criteria and common sense. In addition to analgesics, selected antispasmodics, tranquilizing agents, and even cordotomies may be appropriate.

Infection may be a problem in a number of chronically ill patients; and the treatment, when possible, usually involves the use of an antimicrobial agent. Some patients with chronic bladder infection, such as the paralyzed, may not respond to a potent antibiotic, and it is a curious fact that many may not need them because the hosts sometimes learn to live with their bacteria. Long-term antibiotics in these patients may merely allow the development of resistant strains of bacteria, accomplishing undesirable results like gastrointestinal problems. Hematuria can be troublesome to the extent of requiring transfusions, and it can be particularly difficult if it is secondary to some necessary chemotherapies administered for other malignancies, such as leukemia.

When and if the bladder fills with blood clots, immediate steps must be taken to remove them. Use of catheters is inevitable in these cases, and the catheters themselves may be the cause of severe pain or secondary infection.

Finally, we come to voiding dysfunction. Under certain conditions, timely emptying becomes progressively impaired. The patient may void infrequently, day or night, or may not be able to void at all, or he or she may dribble urine constantly. There is nothing to compare with the smell of stale urine on soiled clothes to galvanize those closest to the patient. While it is always easy to insert an indwelling catheter, other techniques may also be used. Assuming that major surgery cannot be performed, the pharmacologic management of voiding dysfunction can be surprisingly effective. One positive consequence of the Vietnam War is the great amount of basic research conducted on the neuropathic bladder. Thus, many more men and women can now control bladder function (not perfectly but adequately). Drugs are available to make bladders work harder or to relax them and to open and close sphincters. Some investigation on electric stimulation of the bladder or the spinal cord has been done, and the results are not all discouraging. Implantable sphincters are routinely being used today all over the world, and for the most part the surgical risks are quite acceptable since the techniques are not so complicated. Bladder replacements using intestinal segments have been used for years, and the urologic literature constantly reports major and minor innovations in this area.

If, however, these modalities do not work or are impractical, simple collection devices may be used for males. In the case of a male or female, intermittent catheterization, using clean but not necessarily sterile techniques, may be the best choice. Routine intermittent catheterization has been with us for years. This system involves the removal of the indwelling catheter and catheterizing the patient at intervals that are determined by the amount of residual bladder urine left after the patient's best efforts at emptying. Any technique, such as manual expression of bladder contents, use of trigger stimulating points, or drugs, is used to allow noninstrumented emptying, and a record is kept to monitor the patient's progress, if any. Performed gently, intermittent catheterization can be employed indefinitely to the patient's unquestioned benefit. Many patients catheterize themselves after proper instruction, or a family member may be called upon to perform this task. In all cases, whether in a hospital, nursing home, or patient's home, this is almost always preferable to an indwelling catheter. Unfortunately, most hospitals do not have the personnel to perform this service routinely, and the Foley catheter is considered more a staff convenience than a preferred mode of management. There is, in any case, one category of patient in whom a Foley is virtually mandatory, and this is the incontinent female with a small bladder that cannot be made to hold significant amounts of urine. Other than diapering, I know of no other nonsurgical method of management in that particular situation.

By definition, chronic lower tract diseases are of a long-standing, perhaps unremitting, nature. If the process is a bladder or prostate malignancy and cure is beyond reach, the goal of management should be patient comfort and improvement, i.e. quality of life. If the problem is calculi, surgery, when possible, is always successful. In most cases, this can be performed transurethrally, using electronic devices that shatter the stone and leave only small fragments, which can be irrigated from the bladder. If surgery cannot be performed, continuous irrigation may dissolve the stone, but this can take considerable time, even weeks. With certain kinds of stones, complete dissolution may follow alkalinization, hydration, and use of such drugs as allopurinal.

If the problem is a simple enlargement, we may consider limited surgery and look to the research laboratories for development of safe chemical agents that will shrink the prostate. If the problem is neurological, the whole subspecialty of urodynamics has been made available to help define the problem. We often find that one organ failure affects another. So is the case with contributing factors, such as constipation or skin decubiti, the correction of which may assist bladder function. If the problem is the result of general debilitation, some responsible professional must see that whatever can be done is done. It is not hard to understand that neglect affects individuals of any age.

The third category that affects ideal management is the sex and age of the patient. I would like to stress that female patients with chronic lower urinary tract disease, especially the paralyzed, are uniquely victimized. Unfair though it may be, society is particularly intolerant of incontinent females, perhaps because a higher standard of hygiene is expected of females. Then there are the aged, not those who are vigorous but those who are weakened by other disease states that leave them relatively helpless. Some help is almost always necessary with these patients. When available, family members are ideal, but they may not be able to assist over the long term. A visiting nurse service may help, but in the case of the seriously disabled, an indwelling catheter changed at two- to three-week intervals, with suppressant antibacterials, may be the best practical solution.

Ideal management of these patients also depends on resources available. The final word on this should be made by an economist. Although I believe I know what constitutes good care for those patients chronically disabled by urological disease, I am not alone in admitting that I do not know how it should be paid for. Good care costs a great deal, and most people cannot handle these bills unaided. Insurance companies are becoming increasingly unable to pay for all we would like to provide. In fact, they are becoming almost hostile. Even the most sanguine politicians are accepting the notion that the government may also not be able to pay for all the services required.

It has been reported that in one year the total estimated cost of intravenous pyelograms performed prior to transurethral resection of the prostate was as much as $75 million; $28 million of that went for the x-rays, which varied in price from $77 to $125. Of the total, $800,000 was for the kit to prepare patients for the IVP. For this $75 million expenditure we are involved in only one problem, one indication, for one very common procedure in urology.

What are we to do? We must all obviously look for new solutions, new ways of grouping patients, and more cost-effective ways of providing the personnel for the kind of care our patients require while still offering the dignity we would like provided for ourselves and our families. A perfect solution is, obviously, never going to be with us, but the problem is immediate and grave.

Chapter 15

PSYCHOSOCIAL ASPECTS OF THE RADIOTHERAPEUTIC MANAGEMENT OF UROGENITAL MALIGNANCY

JEROME J. SPUNBERG AND SUCHA O. ASBELL

UROGENITAL malignancy is one of the most difficult for the physician. It involves an area that is frequently embarrassing for the patient to discuss; it produces stressful symptoms and in its later stages can be totally incapacitating. Moreover, unlike many other areas of the body, the progress of treatment for cancer in that region is difficult to assess and even more difficult to explain to the patient. Response may be gradual or incomplete. Since a prostatic tumor may take three to six months to regress, the size of the gland does not show the effect of radiation therapy during the treatment course. Similarly, bladder tumors cannot be seen except at the initial or follow-up cystoscopies. If the patient is experiencing increasing urinary frequency secondary to bladder irritation from irradiation, he may choose not to continue daily treatment lacking the immediate gratification of reduction of tumor mass or relief of symptoms. It is the role of the radiation oncologist to encourage and assist patients through the trying times of treatment when there is no ability to visualize the diminution in tumor bulk.

The paradox in the treatment of patients with genitourinary cancer is that those most likely to benefit from radiation therapy (in the short-term relief of their presenting symptoms of pain, hematuria, or loss of neurologic function) are the ones with the worst long-term prognosis, while those with the best prognosis for cure are likely to have few presenting symptoms and demonstrate few beneficial effects of the radiation therapy during the treatment course itself.

The role of radiation therapy in providing relief for the unpleasant and distressing symptoms caused by genitourinary malignancies of the prostate, bladder, kidney, and ureter sites follows.

The Prostate

Cancer of the prostate is divided into four stages utilizing the conventional American system. Early carcinoma is often incidentally detected; more advanced tumors are diagnosed by the increasing size of the prostate gland itself and consequent symptoms until the disease eventually extends beyond the prostate and causes symptoms in distant sites, the so-called metastatic phase.

The patient with early disease may be managed primarily with surgery or radiation therapy. Frequently, the decision to receive one form of therapy or another is dependent upon the patient's psychological status and need to maintain sexual potency since external radiation yields only a 30 percent probability of impotency in contrast to nearly 100 percent with surgery. Interstitial implantation techniques allow even greater sparing of sexual function but require hospitalization and surgical intervention as well. Patients who choose radiation therapy for those reasons are more easily managed during the course of treatment since they are more certain of their decision, whereas other patients to whom radiation therapy has been suggested as primary management must be convinced repetitively of the ability of radiation to cure or control their disease.

One of the most frustrating aspects of early tumor management is that the tumor usually grows slowly after presentation unless it is a poorly differentiated carcinoma. It also regresses slowly, and the patient who chronically asks the physician about his response to therapy is left with little gratification. Patients with relatively early disease, either Stages A or B, have the best prognosis, and with therapy have a minimum five-year survival of approximately 70 percent. In contradistinction, the patient with Stage C disease, where the tumor has spread outside the prostate gland to the periprostatic tissues, has reduced chances of cure. At this point, surgery is of little value as a curative technique and the anticipated five-year survival is only 40 percent with radiation alone.

The most difficult patients to manage, however, are those with metastatic cancer of the prostate. Their problems are multiple and diverse. Unfortunately, this is the most common stage of presentation to the general practitioner, urologist, or radiation therapist. These patients who frequently appear for the first time with widely spread disease in lymph nodes, bones or bone marrow, liver, lungs, or other sites have local symptoms with typical urologic complaints of frequency, urgency, nocturia, dribbling, or obstruction of flow, and also bone pain, renal failure with associated nausea or vomiting, or bone marrow failure with weakness and anemia. Sometimes they present with neurologic deficit as their manifestation of disease only to find at the time of a surgical procedure that the process is due to metastatic prostate cancer.

It is imperative that the radiation therapist anticipate the various symptoms and problems of patients with metastatic cancer and explain these to the patient so that, should these occur, he is prepared to make quick and appropriate judgments and take immediate action to prevent life-threatening processes from proceeding. It is our practice to inform the patient about potential symptoms of epidural metastasis, both in a cervical or thoracolumbar region, so that if weakness or paresthesia appears, he reports them immediately to avoid the catastrophic possibility of paraplegia. If paraplegia sets in, the condition is usually irreversible with added radiation alone.

We as radiation therapists also advise our patients of the importance of frequent intravenous pyelograms to assess renal function. Since their bone pain may not be severe or life-threatening and since hormonal management is instituted, the patients feel that their condition is being stabilized. However, silent growth of the prostate superiorly out of the prostatic bed into surrounding tissues may gradually obstruct the ureters and be unknown to the examining physician because such extension is usually not palpable. The result could be ureteral obstruction and subsequent renal shutdown.

A stressful aspect of tumors and of prostate cancer is the hormonal management that may be prescribed simultaneously or in sequence with radiation therapy. It may also be necessary to treat a patient prophylactically to the breasts to avoid embarrassing gynecomastia and unpleasant gynecodynia. If, however, we have not had the opportunity to see a patient early in the course of his estrogen therapy, it is too late to help avert these symptoms and we are faced with a man disturbed by apparent loss of masculinity through voice change and by a more feminine appearance from enlarging breasts. These problems compound the intricate management of the patient with more advanced prostatic cancer.

The radiation oncologist has much to offer the patient with metastatic disease by giving quality survival. Frequent examinations allow for the management of anemia, pain, urologic, or neurologic dysfunction. Patients not previously placed on hormones might return in follow-up examination with progressing disease and thus alert the urologist to the need for possible orchiectomy or administration of estrogens. It is important to advise patients that although their survival rate is diminished from metastatic disease, their quality of survival can be maintained with appropriate radiation therapy. Since prostatic tumors are slow growing and metastases can occur over a long period of time, patients have to live with their disease and understand the chronic nature of their condition. They require assurance and alleviation of fears about surviving with unrelieved discomfort. The largest psychological handle that can be given is to provide continuing hope for management by never offering an exact estimate of longevity. An attitude should be generated by the radiation oncologists and community that each day is important and should be enjoyed to the fullest. Each day should be utilized in living, not in dying. The radiation therapist must emphasize to the patient that he has a chronic disease not altogether different from other chronic diseases, such as diabetes, heart disease, or rheumatoid arthritis but with the advantage that a normal life style can frequently be maintained with only occasional intervention from the physician, as opposed to chronic hospitalization and physician intervention.

In treating carcinoma of the prostate, in either early or late manifestations of disease, radiation therapists offer both a physical and psychological support system for their patients.

The Bladder

As with prostatic cancer, bladder cancer is also staged A through D by an American system, with stage D representing distant metastatic disease. Patients presenting to the radiation therapy department frequently have more advanced stages, since these are the ones most amenable to management with this modality. The combination of radiation therapy and surgery is frequently utilized in this disease. Thus, the management of patients with ostomies must be preplanned and psychological preparation provided for extended survival with an ostomy. Since cancer of the urinary bladder is usually a locally aggressive transitional cell carcinoma and tends not to protract over long periods of time as for patients with prostatic metastatic disease, patient management is more often directed toward local control rather than chronic illness and expected slow demise.

Pain, frequency, urgency, and hematuria are the most common presenting symptoms. The radiation therapy may ameliorate the hematuria, but the frequency and urgency that accompany the process do not disappear as treatment continues. Instead, they may be exacerbated or exaggerated. Radiation itself is an irritating phenomenon that makes it difficult for patients to accept treatment. Patients require continuous reassurance and support that at the conclusion of therapy these symptoms will regress. Once again, there is no visible tumor for the radiation therapist to follow, and usually no palpable tumor. Thus, it is difficult to reassure the patients of benefit, especially when the only manifestations of therapy are those of annoying side effects.

Preoperative radiation therapy followed by cystectomy is often the best alternative for control of the cancer locally. Unfortunately, all too often the patient becomes manipulative during his course of therapy, attempting to extract from the radiation therapist a change of plan that would eliminate the surgical component upon completion of the radiation portion. Basically, the fear of surgery may begin to outweigh the fear of the cancer itself once radiation therapy has provided some relief, and it becomes challenging to make the patient comprehend why combination therapy is better than radiation alone.

For patients who are not able to undergo a surgical procedure or who have refused surgery, radiation alone may be utilized as the sole curative attempt. This requires a treatment course of seven to ten weeks in some cases and increases the risks of radiation side effects and long-term complications such as chronic cystitis, pelvic fibrosis, contracted bladder, or fistula formation. Many of these side effects can be managed medically without surgical intervention but must be fully explained in advance to the patient. By careful treatment planning using recent tools such as the computerized axial tomography (CAT) scanner, side effects can generally be minimized or avoided completely.

Carcinoma of the bladder may metastasize to soft tissue or bone.

Any site of metastatic disease is amenable to radiation palliation. Although newer chemotherapeutic agents are being introduced to assist in the management of metastatic disease, radiation remains the prime source for pain control. The failure to control the disease locally in the pelvis with any modality is much more likely to produce distressing symptoms for the patient and result in eventual demise than metastases in bladder cancer.

The Kidney and Ureter

Radiation therapy is involved in the frequent postoperative management and occasional preoperative management of renal carcinoma. Generally, however, our role has been more traditionally utilized in the management of metastatic disease where (because this is a relatively radio-resistant tumor) slightly higher doses are required for palliation. Partial or total relief from pain or bleeding may be anticipated in most cases. These patients may survive for many years after their initial surgery and their time of demise is unpredictable. Therapeutic management must be contemplated with longevity in mind.

Conclusion

Radiation therapy has an important role in both the curative and palliative management of urogenital malignancy. In bladder tumors, the focus is on local control of symptoms within the pelvis. In cancer of the kidney and ureter, radiation is generally utilized more for distant metastases or recurrence. In prostate cancer, both local and distant disease are common causes for referral to the radiation therapy department.

Radiation is used alone or in combination with other modalities, such as surgery or chemotherapy. Since there are few chemotherapeutic agents with high probability of killing tumor cells and since many patients are too old or the disease too advanced for surgical attempts, radiation therapy has remained an essential ingredient in total management over the years. Radiation therapy serves in palliation of pain, urologic symptoms, secondary neurologic symptoms, and orthopedic symptoms from metastases, as well as in initial curative efforts and long-term follow-up.

New anticipated approaches will include different fractionation schemes of radiation, combination with chemotherapeutic agents, radiation protectors and sensitizers, implantation techniques, and improved surgical methods. However, in the management of malignancy in this most personal and sensitive region of the body, the provision of a psychological support system for the patient will remain the key to success on a long- or short-term basis.

Chapter 16

DIABETES, IMPOTENCE, AND SEXUALITY

Arnold Melman

ONE of the problems with sexuality and sexual dysfunction is that many of the people who talk and write about the subject do so in an anecdotal way. Surgeons, who have to make difficult decisions about what to do for people, like to have numbers and to make plans on an objective basis. Here, I have objectively defined some of the psychologic problems of people who have diabetes and impotence. In recent months we have operated on a small group who had impotence so severe that they required penile prostheses.

The penis has areas of connective tissue, smooth muscle, and spongy spaces that fill with blood during an erection. It takes from 30 to 60 milliliters of blood during an increase in the blood flow to cause an erection. We are not sure if the blood flow increases and stays at an increased rate or if the blood flow increases and becomes trapped in the penis to be released during detumescence. Many veins exit from both the dorsal and ventral portions of the penis. During transsexual surgery, when the veins are clamped, an erection can actually be created. There are many veins draining from the ventral aspect of the tissue that probably are more important than the dorsal veins in blood flow within the erectile tissue of the penis.

There is a profound neural innovation to the penis mostly passing behind the inferior and lateral aspect of the prostate, and that is the problem. When we do radical surgery on the prostate, we destroy those nerves; when we do radical surgery on the rectum, we also distort them. If we do radical bladder surgery, we destroy the nerves, with over 90 percent of the patients becoming impotent.

Since erection is a dilatation of the arterial inflow to these spongy spaces, when the inflow resistance is less than the outflow resistance, an erection occurs. Detumescence will occur when the inflow resistance becomes higher than the outflow; the penis then will empty the increased blood.

Erection is multifaceted since the brain and spinal cord are also necessary for function. Overlying and probably governing all three factors are hormones. Again, there is much we do not know. We do not know the effect of testosterone upon the erectile tissue of the penis, for example. We know that if we castrate a man because of carcinoma of the prostate, the penis will shrink. And we know that during puberty phallic enlargement occurs. Testosterone has some effect on the erectile tissue, but we do not know the details. There have been studies of castration (in Norway where they used to castrate sex offenders) showing that for years afterward the subjects were able to have an erection; the exact interplay is uncertain. It is certain that if one stimulates the forebrain (a portion of the cortex) in monkeys, they have an erection. Erection is a reflex event; you cannot will an erection.

There is a 50 percent incidence of impotence in diabetics. It had been thought that no relationship exists between impotence and the severity or duration of the disease. However, a few reports state that among diabetic young men who go into ketoacidosis, impotence is relieved when ketoacidosis is treated. Thus, diabetes control probably is important. In the United States, there are 5 million diabetic men, 2½ million of whom are potentially impotent. Impotence presents as the initial clinical manifestation for about 13 to 20 percent of the diabetic men. Despite loss of ability to have erection, nothing happens to the libido. The patients want to be able to have genital intercourse. They can have ejaculation and orgasm but are not able to achieve vaginal penetration and become frustrated.

We have looked at the effects of diabetes upon the nerve transmitters that control the blood vessels in the erectile tissue. The principal neurotransmitter of the vascular smooth muscle of blood vessels is norepinephrine, or noradrenalin. That substance is stored in the nerve endings next to the muscle tissue itself. We remove that tissue and measure the norepinephrine of many of the men we have operated on to implant penile prostheses, e.g. transsexuals and men who have had penectomies because of cancer of the penis. In normal men, there are 880 picograms of norepinephrine per milligram of tissue, about eight times higher than in muscle itself. In men who are impotent and diabetic and who have taken insulin, concentration of norepinephrine is one-eighth the normal amount. In diabetics whose illness is less severe and controlled by diet, there are significantly reduced levels of norepinephrine, but a bit less than that of the men on insulin.

Since 1863, when Von Eckhardt stimulated the nervi erigenti in the dog and considered that a parasympathetic nerve, it has been taught that the parasympathetic nervous system is predominantly responsible for erection. We have decided to question this theory. We measured the enzyme in the erectile tissue responsible for acetylcholine production (acetylcholine is the substance released by the parasympathetic nerve that causes its effect) and discovered that there was no activity of acetylcholine in erectile tissue in any patient, including normal people. We concluded that the parasympathetic nervous system, at least within the level of the corporal bodies themselves, probably is not important and that the sympathetic nervous system is the more significant of the two. There are recent manuscripts that seem to substantiate this finding.

One factor influencing our decision whether or not to implant penile prostheses in patients is that if people are impotent because they do not get along with their wives or their sex partners, this is a symptom of their marital or related problems, and they use it as an excuse. Even if a penile prosthesis is put in that kind of patient, he won't be happy.

We have to be very careful in selecting patients. That is why patients are sent to sleep lab (to test tumescence) and to a psychiatrist. Any surgeon who has performed a radical cystectomy knows why a man is impotent. But with diabetes, the individual may be impotent because of neurologic dysfunction as a result of diabetes; or (as suggested earlier) he may be diabetic, depressed, or not getting along with his wife but not truly be impotent on a disease basis.

If a diabetic man tells us he is impotent, how do we evaluate the patient until we get his tissue and measure norepinephrine or do the nocturnal tumescence study? Can we use a psychologic screen? A sexual functioning index developed at Johns Hopkins has been used for this purpose. The test is a 250-question self-assessment exam of ten phases of current sexual function. A man or woman is asked to evaluate personal sexual functioning—how he or she thinks it is.

What did we find? We compared the results of five patients who had been operated on and who had organic impotence. The normal was about 213, and these five patients got a *total* score of about 501—clearly a difference.

We seemed to find specifically that the role, symptoms, and affects were low compared to the Johns Hopkins subjects who had sexual dysfunction. These studies have not as yet separated psychogenic and organic impotence although they have noted that the role and affect areas are particularly important in differentiating people who are impotent from the normal. We need more patients to distinguish between the organic and the psychogenic. The impotent man tends to become more feminine in his outlook and responses as he is less able to satisfy his wife with genital sex. The psychology literature reports that one probable cause of psychogenic impotence is affect: depression and guilt. Our five patients with demonstrated organic impotence seemed to have very high levels of anxiety, depression, guilt, and hostility.

I have done about eighty penile prosthesis operations through the penis because the incision cannot be seen and there is better control in dilating the corporum. One of my patients is a forty-two-year-old engineer. He had been seeing a psychiatrist for five years. He was on forty units a day of NPH insulin and had a psychologic depression. No one had told him about diabetic impotence. He could not satisfy his wife; his marriage was going to pot, and he was having trouble with his work.

I implanted the prosthesis in this patient. Usually, I have patients wait about six weeks after prosthesis insertion to tell them they can have intercourse. After about three weeks, I called my patient and spoke with his wife on the telephone. She was giggling and obviously having a grand time at home. The operation had clearly changed their marriage.

I have placed the inflatable penile prosthesis. This is an excellent operation with about a 5 percent mechanical breakdown rate. It gives a little firmer erection. The prosthesis itself costs $1,600, and in certain areas the insurance companies will not cover the cost. I give patients a choice of prosthesis after telling them the pros and cons of both prostheses. If they ask me for my opinion, I suggest the Small-Carrion for the older, sicker, more frail patient. For a younger, more vigorous patient who may change clothes in a locker-room, I suggest the inflatable penile prosthesis.

I have discussed impotence with a group of spinal cord injured patients. They were quick to remind me to always tell patients that genital intercourse is not the only way to experience sex. It is important to counsel patients before insertion of a penile prosthesis. People like to insist that genital intercourse is the only way for them; they don't enjoy having oral-genital sex, using stimulators, vibrators, or dildos. But it is a duty of the surgeon to discuss alternatives with patients before they make their decisions.

Chapter 17

MECHANICAL ASPECTS OF RESTORATION OF SEXUAL FUNCTION IN THE DISABLED MALE PATIENT

JAMES F. GLENN

ALTHOUGH this subject would not have been openly discussed ten or fifteen years ago, except by a very brave few, today urologic surgeons accept the responsibility for restoration of normal sexual function in the disabled male patient. The first surgical efforts began with the availability of a very primitive penile prosthesis, the Pearman prosthesis, an acrylic rod that was implanted beneath the fascia of the penile shaft. Frequent complications with this device often necessitated its removal and made it most unsatisfactory. To avoid the erosion and infection from this type of implant, some investigators suggested a device that could be put inside the corpora, but others felt that this also was an invitation to disaster. Time proved that this was possible, and the most effective penile prosthesis ever devised was developed. Everything else that has followed, with the exception of the inflation device, has been derived from that early Small-Carrion prosthesis.

Our group began seriously implanting these modern devices almost a decade ago and by April 1, 1980, had implanted 187. We have reported on the first seventy-six of these implanted devices, recognizing their complications as well as the advantages gained in their use.

The device has been implanted in diabetic patients, in those suffering traumatic paraplegia, in patients suffering priapism from all causes, especially young black males who have priapism as a consequence of sickle cell disease in their adolescence. We have implanted the device in patients on dialysis who, for one reason or another, have never been candidates for transplantation, and we have implanted the device in patients who have been successfully transplanted but who have failed to regain satisfactory potency.

Only rarely have we implanted the device truly for psychological reasons. This may be contrary to general experience around the country, but we have felt uneasy in undertaking a major surgical effort, that of implanting a foreign body with all of its attendant complications, in someone who has a fundamental psychological or psychiatric problem. On a few occasions, we have done this at the absolute insistence of friends in psychology, but it is not common practice.

We have implanted in patients with demyelinating diseases and a broad spectrum of other disabled people, but the overwhelming number of patients who have been implanted are those with malignant disease. Predominantly, these have been prostate cancer and bladder cancer patients, but we have also implanted patients who have undergone radical abdominal peritoneal surgery for colon cancer as well.

There are numerous complications accompanying implantation. Principally, these involve infection of the prosthesis to such an extent that removal is necessary. We have seen massive sloughs of the genitalia as a consequence of this on two occasions. One patient who extruded both of his prostheses through the urethra simply pulled them out of the urethral meatus. On other occasions, we have had to remove the prosthesis because of pain from an unknown source. However, removal of the prosthesis in these patients caused immediate cessation of the discomfort. Although this discomfort, a burning perineal sensation, was thought to be from pudendal nerve irritation, pudendal nerve injection and various other maneuvers for its relief proved to be unsuccessful.

If the implanted device is too small, the distal portion of the penis droops, and it has been necessary to reoperate on these patients to insert a larger device. As another major operation, this clearly is also a complication.

If the above sounds discouraging, it should be remembered that impotency is a most stressful reality. The urologist sees a large number of cancer patients who are potentially sexually disabled by malignant disease. Approximately 13 percent of all cancers are those of the lower genitourinary system, all of which would potentially disable the patient sexually. This is a formidable group of patients, with malignant disease that is amenable to surgical cure or palliation that threatens the sexual viability of the individual. Five-year survival rates are important factors because we must recognize that the restoration of normal function is dependent upon the population for whom this survival rate is applicable. This population increases as we steadily increase our cure rate. With this improving cure rate, many urologists have accepted the challenge to proceed to restore sexual function once the patient is deemed to be a potential cure. In recent years, we have not felt it necessary to wait to see if the patient is cured because, in the prostate cancer or bladder cancer patient, this might mean a period of four, five, or six years. In our opinion, there is little rationale behind condemning a patient to impotence and sexual debility during that interval. Therefore, in general, we have considered a patient a candidate for penile prosthesis as early as six months after radial cystoprostatectomy or radical cystectomy. On the average, the implant is done about one year after the original surgery. Of course, some patients are potent after radical prostatectomy or radical cystectomy; others must be screened for psychological impotence in the absence of a surgical history.

The screening device currently being used is the penile tumescence monitor. This is used at the bedside in the patient's private room. The sensors or loops are placed about the penis with one at its base and the other subcoronally for monitoring nocturnal tumescence. The backside of the apparatus is concealed from the patient. The normal male will have three or four sustained erections during sleep on any given night, and this erectile activity is recorded on a graph. In recording the number of events, the duration of each event, and the acceptable tracing quality, we can predict the reproducibility of tumescence and, thus, determine whether the patient has true organic impotence. Patients who complain of surgical organic impotence are not always subjected to this testing as we accept them at their word. Recognizing the importance of any information in this regard to both the patient and his wife, we discuss every possible factor with them before proceeding.

Following the development of the Small–Carrion prosthesis came the development of the inflatable device. This has inflatable balloons that are connected to a pump that pumps fluid in and out of the ballons from a reservoir. The storage reservoir is installed under the abdominal wall, with the pump device usually implanted on the right side of the upper part of the scrotum. The device itself is in the corpora cavernosa. Clearly, there can be problems arising from this type of implant also. Most of these are mechanical: The pump can go bad; the valve can become defective; the small connectors can become defective; the tubing can become dislodged; the reservoir can leak; and fluid can be expelled. However, these complications have been worked on, and the device is at least 90 percent reliable.

Patients are in the hospital for about six days for antibiotic therapy and implantation. On discharge, they are admonished not to manipulate the pump. After six weeks, they return to the office and we teach them how to squeeze the pump for inflation and for deflation.

The correction of male impotence as a result of malignant disease is established as a reasonable procedure. The only departure I would take from accepted urologic practice is that we perform this procedure earlier. There is no reason to condemn a patient to disability for a long period while we wait around to see whether or not he is going to have recurrent disease, particularly in view of the fact that recurrence of prostate cancer is not a death warrant. Recurrence of prostatic cancer can be treated hormonally, chemotherapeutically, and radiologically. With bladder cancer there is hope that chemotherapeutic agents and even immunal therapy can offer even further advantages in control of the malignant disease. As a consequence, I believe that we need not be timid in approaching a patient for surgical correction of impotence.

Chapter 18

THE DEPARTING GERIATRIC PATIENT

Hans H. Zinsser

AS the individual ages, some of his immunological competence fades. As a result, cancers of the pancreas and prostate have become very important causes of death in the last three decades. Since our knowledge regarding cardiovascular disease is improving, these two cancers may turn out to be leading causes of death in the geriatric patient.

The older patient is no better prepared for death from cancer than the younger patient. In fact, many elderly people assume a cloak of invincibility, having survived so much longer than most of their contemporaries. This state of mind is a cause of great depression when a final diagnosis of terminal cancer is arrived at. The older patient still craves as acutely for affection and, indeed, for sexual contact as a younger patient, and so he clings to continuing life.

How can the emotional problems of the elderly in this situation be managed? In many instances, we cannot in truthfulness say that we believe the patient will die of cancer. So many other conditions can coexist in the elderly patient with prostatic cancer, for instance, that cardiovascular disease may kill many more patients than the cancer itself. Whether this is in part because of the hormonal control of both cardiovascular disease and of prostatic tumor growth is difficult to say, but it raises the point that we cannot with the same assurance say to the geriatric cancer patient that he is going to die of his tumor as we can to the younger patient not at risk from other conditions. We are, of course, forced to inform someone in the cancer patient's family of the presence of tumor. However, we may not necessarily have to risk exacerbating the depression of an already somewhat confused and perhaps depressed elderly patient with a blunt statement that he has a cancer that will kill him.

The geriatric patient may have some difficulty comprehending the nature of his disease, just as he may be somewhat confused about the state of the world in general. It is unlikely that patients with severe, organic brain damage should be apprised of their cancerous condition at all.

There are some cancers that are so well controlled by hormonal or other chemotherapeutic modes of therapy that we may safely shift to the side of underinforming the victim of his true condition. On the other hand, as people grow older their responsibilities may be overwhelming, necessitating a longer advance notice of their impending mortality than patients in a younger age group.

We know, in general, that the older the patient, the more slowly the cancer progression. Likewise, the usefulness of radiation therapy in the older patient is likely to be considerably less. Until more is known about specific chemotherapeutic modalities, we must be alert for the greater incidence of side effects following chemotherapy in the geriatric patient. A young person might afford for instance to bleed or to undergo transient bacteriemia. The older patient may not be able to survive such a circulatory assault.

Our approach to the geriatric patient already under custodial care who develops an acute presenting illness, such as urinary retention secondary to prostatic cancer, must of course depend on a tissue diagnosis for future management. The considerations for biopsy in the older patient are merely that we are inclined to settle for less tissue and less trauma the older the patient gets. This makes me favor needle biopsy of the prostate rather than a punch biopsy, because of the lower morbidity due to bleeding or urinary leakage. With the elegance of fiber-optic equipment available, the diagnosis of pancreatic cancer can be done earlier than before and the lesion may even eventually be biopsied endoscopically. In many instances, the patient should not have any radical surgery. Contrary to some expectations, the geriatric patient has no higher threshold for pain than his younger counterpart, but the margin between effective pain medication and toxicity is a much narrower one in the older patient. Just as in pediatrics it is said that a child is not a little man, so in turn the geriatric person is not just a slightly older fellow. Much pharmacology is radically altered by the passage of time, and the patient in his eighties and nineties can occasionally be handled with fractional doses of many medications.

We must anticipate that renal, pancreatic, pituitary, and even adrenal cortical function may be much diminished in these older patients, and that too rapid replacement of these missing materials may be deleterious to patient management. The caloric requirements of the older patient are sometimes considerably reduced in relation to his more active younger counterpart.

In many of these patients, bladder neck obstruction unrelated to cancer may coexist with other diseases, and one should be careful not to ignore such an eventuality when utilizing agents that may affect both renal function and urinary output. It is axiomatic that when it is inevitable that the patient, because of the nature of his cancer, realizes that a lump or a malfunction has recurred, one must place effort on the reassurance that there are effective palliative procedures that are being pursued as actively as possible. The palliative procedures should be explained in full to the patient, and he should be made an active judge about the efficacy of each step of the palliation. He too will be in a position to evaluate what each step of the therapy has accomplished, and can be actively involved as much as or more than the paramedical personnel required to keep the terminal care period as long as necessary.

There is a continuing and extending body of opinion that feels that beyond a certain age heroic measures should not be carried out to retain life. The crux of this debate would seem to be whether the patient is deriving pleasure from or even knowledge of the world around him. With the geriatric patient, the pressure of obtaining his organs for transplantation is rarely a consideration; most organs have already served their time and would probably be of little value to someone else. Perhaps this is not true of the cornea of the eye. In some pathology departments, all eyes are harvested at autopsy. The patient's family should be warned about this.

The degree of vanity and precision of body image of the older patient cannot be overemphasized. A palliative device or contrivance, which in the younger patient might be readily adopted and accommodated, might be a massive blow to the dignity of the older man or woman. I think specifically about one patient who underwent a hysterectomy without any feeling of loss of dignity or womanhood, but for whom proffered removal of her bladder and the setting up of an external contrivance to collect urine were major deterrents to allowing the surgeons to treat her bladder tumor with the hope of cure.

Another consideration in the care of the terminal geriatric patient is that the older the patient, the older his doctor is likely to be. This is rarely true of the paramedical personnel, most of whom have retired by the time they reach the age of the patient. The older doctor, however, tends to minimize the symptoms of the cancer patient because he too has aches and pains in the joints, dyspepsia with meals, and may himself have weathered several serious illnesses.

This correlation of symptoms in the doctor and in the patient tends to make the physician far less involved emotionally with specific aspects of the patient's disease, but by no means is it any easier for him to see the patient, perhaps a life-long friend, die.

Chapter 19

ANTICIPATORY GRIEVING AND COGNITIVE MASTERY IN THE MANAGEMENT OF THE PSYCHOLOGICAL ASPECTS OF KIDNEY REJECTION

REGE SZUTS STEWART

THE stress of kidney rejection is accompanied by complex psychological reactions. Depression is the most common psychologic reaction to dialysis whether secondary to native kidney failure or to rejection (Stewart and Stewart, 1979). Abram and Buchanan have observed that suicidal behavior often occurs when the patient is placed back on dialysis following rejection (1976; 1977). This is an understandable phenomenon when one realizes that the transplanted kidney is a highly cachected object, which offers the hope of returning to normal life free of dialysis. As Kemph and Bermann (1969) have demonstrated, fantasies of rebirth are common themes among recipients.

Thus, a functioning graft becomes the symbol of improved quality of life, a new beginning free of the problems of dialysis. It is no wonder that the loss of function in this highly valued organ is accompanied by depression. The patient mourns not just the loss of the kidney but also his hope for a productive life. He is also faced with the possibility of death. The ensuing depression may interfere with the patient's ability to return to dialysis and may even effect the frequency and severity of medical complications. Eisendrath (1969) has presented compelling data indicating that severe depression accompanied by a sense of helplessness and hopelessness may effect the severity of medical complications and result in death. Accordingly, the primary prevention and prompt treatment of depression becomes a very important task. We need to understand the stages recipients experience before we discuss treatment. Reichsman had already outlined the stages patients experience on dialysis (1972), and this chapter will attempt to describe the psychological stages involved in transplantation and the techniques of primary prevention.

Psychological Stages of Kidney Transplant Rejection

Optimistic Anticipation

Once plans are made for renal transplant, patients await surgery eagerly. During this stage, optimism prevails and patients display a high level of denial. As mentioned earlier, there is a fantasy of renewed health and the hope of a productive life. Patients often are reluctant to discuss the possibility of rejection. They listen politely when possibility of rejection or other medical complication is raised and assure the interviewer that this will not happen to them. A certain amount of denial may have a protective function, for it prevents the patient from being overwhelmed by anxiety. Studies of cardiac patients have indicated that those with some level of denial did better than those who felt pessimistic about their chance for survival. On the other hand, denial may be of pathologic proportions; some patients will refuse to even consider the possibility of complications. As one twenty-year-old man stated: "Don't talk to me about complications, talk to my mother. She does all the worrying for me." Denial is a defense against overwhelming anxiety and the unconscious fear that surgery may not be successful. When there is a breakdown of the denial, intense anxiety will surface.

Apprehensive Waiting

This stage starts immediately following surgery and lasts until rejection occurs. The prevailing mood is anxiety and irritability. Often, the mood corresponds to the creatinine level and urine output of the day. Our patients are aware of their daily values. Drop in creatinine is accompanied with relief and optimistic outlook, while a rise results in irritability, demanding behavior, and depression. If rejection does not occur within the first month, most patients' anxiety levels wane, but do not completely disappear. Fear of rejection persists even in patients who have done well three or more years out of transplant. In a way, however, a certain amount of this fear is important so that the patient will take his immunosuppressants. When this concern is not present, the patient may stop medication, and this can result in transplant rejection.

Rejection Grief

The majority of initial rejections are reversible and most patients are aware of this. The fulminating rejection is usually the only one which cannot be arrested or reversed initially. Most patients will experience several rejections before losing their kidney and the time period is variable lasting from within a week of surgery until several years after.

Most patients who experience their first rejection will use the mechanism of denial. They will try to minimize or rationalize their symptoms, and express the hope that this is only a temporary setback. Once irreversible rejection is established, patients experience anger and depression. The severity of psychological reaction seems to be influenced by the patient's age, the length of graft survival, available family support, and the patient's own coping mechanism. In general, patients who had functioning grafts for over a year and who have a reasonably good prognosis for a second graft will do better. Patients whose graft either never functioned or who developed severe medical complications in conjunction with their rejection will experience severe depression. The depression may be accompanied by acting out, negatives, and (in younger patients) refusal to follow medical advice. This reaction often results in the alienation of both family and nursing staff and thus in a greater sense of hopelessness and helplessness.

Acceptance of Rejection and Dialysis

Gradually, the acute depression is replaced by resignation and acceptance of dialysis. Some patients are more willing to accept dialysis if they have a hope for another transplant. This is essentially a form of bargaining; the patient promises to return to the rigors of dialysis in hope of eventually receiving a new kidney. Those for whom another transplantation is not a possibility experience recurrent or chronic depressive episodes.

Emotional Parallels of Transplant Rejection and the Dying Patient

The emotions (denial, anger, and depression) experienced by patients whose kidney is rejected parallel those seen in the dying patient, although the sequence can be variable. Anxiety is an extremely common affect in this group of patients, second in importance only to depression. The form of bargaining is also different. The patient whose graft failed has only two choices: death or return to dialysis. During the past three years, not one patient in our center had refused dialysis and consciously chosen death. One can argue that patients who act out and become noncompliant once back on dialysis are unconsciously seeking death. Alternately, the noncompliant behavior can be seen as a form of masked depression.

Primary Prevention

At the University of Texas Health Science Center at Dallas all living related donors and most recipients have psychiatric evaluations. Since our policy is to transplant all medically qualifying recipients who desire a kidney, the emphasis of the psychological evaluation is more on primary prevention of psychological problems than on selecting ideal recipients. If major psychopathology is present in the recipient, supportive psychotherapy is suggested prior to transplantation rather than turning the candidate away. We have allowed patients with borderline personality and major depressive disorders to undergo transplants and thus far these patients have done well. We have no experience with schizophrenic patients.

At the time of the interview, the patient is given a detailed description of the surgery, and is asked to express his reactions to it. For example, I tell the patient that when he wakes up in the recovery room he will have an intravenous device, a nasogastric tube, and a Foley catheter. He will also feel groggy and uncomfortable, although relatively free of pain. I encourage the patient to imagine himself in the recovery room and urge him to describe how he would feel. Well defended, psychologically healthy patients can verbalize their feelings of anxiety, fear, and concern and can master the situation in the office. Patients who are very anxious or who have difficulty dealing with abstract terms will not be able to anticipate their reaction. I tell these patients what the frequent emotional reactions are and ask how they would handle them. Often, the patient is encouraged to explore several ways of dealing with common complications (pain, initial anuria, vomiting, and so forth). Essentially, this is a form of cognitive mastery where the patient can intellectually master hypothetical situations in a relaxed environment without being encumbered by intense anxiety or depression.

The last part of the interview focuses on rejection. The patient is told that most recipients experience some form of rejection within the first month and that most of the first episode is reversible, although about 15 to 20 percent will lose the kidney. Anticipatory grieving is encouraged by the exploration of feelings in anticipation of organ loss. Most patients realize that they will be depressed but probably would go back on dialysis. If the patient states "that couldn't happen to me" or "this kidney has to work," I persist in raising the possibility that it may fail. I always reassure the patient that his physicians will do everything possible to save the kidney. We express the hope that his kidney will not reject, but for sake of completeness, we need to discuss how he would handle a rejection.

After transplant, I see the patient periodically. If rejection does occur, the patient is encouraged to verbalize his feelings. Depression, disappointment, and anger are very common reactions. Later on I start discussing the possibility of dialysis. Usually there is initial protest, but after a week or two of bolus steroid therapies, radiation therapy and some invasive procedures (angiogram, kidney biopsy, etc.), most patients are relieved to leave the hospital and return to dialysis. One patient after his rejection stated, "I was so sure that this wouldn't happen to me" and another stated, "It was easier to handle in your office." Both experienced brief depressions that responded to supportive interviews and returned to dialysis. Lindemann (1944) had observed that grieving relatives who had anticipated the loss of a loved one and had time to accept the impending loss did better than those for whom death was an unexpected event. Thus, the concept of anticipatory grieving is used here in the context of organ loss and in the mastery of resultant depression.

In summary, depression is the usual response to organ rejection. Primary prevention using cognitive mastery and the principles of anticipatory grieving seems to modify both the intensity and length of depression.

References

Abram, S., and Buchanan, D.C.: The gift of life: A review of the psychological aspects of kidney transplantation. *International Journal of Psychiatry in Medicine*, 7, 1976 and 1977.

Eisendrath, R.M.: The role of grief and fear in the death of kidney transplant patients. *American Journal of Psychiatry, 126*:381-387, 1969.

Kemph, Y.P., Bermann, E.A., and Coppolillo, H.P.: Kidney transplant and shifts in family dynamics. *American Journal of Psychiatry, 125*:1495-1490, 1969.

Lindemann, E.: Symptomatology and management of acute grief. *American Journal of Psychiatry, 101*:141-148, 1944.

Reichsman, F., and Levy, N.B.: Problems of adaptation to maintenance hemodialysis. *Archives of Internal Medicine, 130*:859-865, 1972.

Stewart, R.S., and Stewart, R.M.: Psychiatric aspects of chronic renal disease: Hemodialysis and transplantation. *Weekly Psychiatry Update Series, 27*, 1979.

Chapter 20

PSYCHOLOGICAL ASPECTS OF CHRONIC HEMODIALYSIS AND PSYCHIATRIC COMPLICATIONS OF THE PATIENT: A REVIEW OF THE LITERATURE

LINDA M. RHODES

Introduction

THIS chapter is a literature review of the psychosocial aspects of end-stage renal disease and chronic hemodialysis. Theories on chronic illness and the sick role are reviewed from a sociological framework. Biological aspects of the disease as it relates to behavior are presented, as are the psychological reactions and psychiatric complications of patients with end-stage renal disease. The psychiatric complications are presented in two segments: emotional disturbance and stress of the dialysis regimen. Depression, dependency vs. independency conflicts, suicide, and defense mechanisms are those treated under emotional disturbance; the stress of chronic hemodialysis is reported in the areas of body image, threat of death, and family stress. The review concludes with an assessment of the research methods and subject concentration that have been employed by the social sciences to study the psychological aspects of end-stage renal failure patients.

Psychological Aspects of Chronic Hemodialysis: The Patient Theoretical View of the Sick Role

Individuals who utilize chronic hemodialysis will be sick for the rest of their lives unless they receive a transplant. Dialysis patients may feel better but they do not feel well (Abram et al., 1971). Thus, this review begins with a consideration of what it is to be sick. Talcott Parsons (1951) cites four characteristics of the sick role in American culture: there is an exemption from normal social responsibilities; the sick person must be taken care of by others; he or she must want to get well; and the individual must seek technical help to become better. It is the physician who legitimizes the patient as being a sick person. Most often the role is seen as being temporary; thus, the privileges and exemptions of the sick role are short term. Parsons describes these privileges as *secondary gain*. The sick role is achieved negatively; no one should want to get sick. It is important that the sick person not be seen by his caregivers as causing the illness. The patient is not to be at fault, nor feel any guilt for his illness.

A major negative aspect of the sick role is that the sick person is vulnerable for exploitation because he is seen as helpless. The patient lacks the technical competence to cure himself. In an illness state, the individual experiences a degree of impairment, pain, and disequilibrium, which substantiates the perception by others that he is helpless. While the individual is sick, his participation in the social system is always related to his state of illness. The sick role is seen by Parsons as a deviant one. The sick form a subculture; it is, however, a culture that includes the nonsick caregivers. Thus, the sick cannot form a collectivity and, therefore, remain impotent in their sick role.

According to Fox (1959), illness is more than a biological condition; it is also a social role assigned patterned characteristics and requirements. Most of the requirements defined by Fox are similar to the Parsonsian model. There must be some degree of impairment in the ability to carry out normal tasks. The patient is encouraged to withdraw from everyday activity. While an individual is not held morally acountable for being sick, the patient is expected to seek competent help and to dutifully follow the advice offered by the source of that help, his doctor.

Illness also causes a disturbance in the psychological and social functioning of the individual. When the illness is a serious one, the ordinary patterns of social existence are greatly modified. A man who is sick must adapt to a new world of sickness, hospitals, doctors, and patients.

Chronically ill people often experience an *identity spread* (Strauss and Glaser, 1975). Other people assume that the sick person cannot act, work, or be normal. The presentation of the sick self greatly affects one's sense of self-identity. The instability in the social role caused by the disease feeds back to the sick person's image of himself. It means that he must readjust previous relationships, cope with the stigmas attributed to his disease, and convince others that he is normal. Nonsick persons tend to overgeneralize the sick person's visible symptoms, which dominate the interaction.

A general problem faced by the chronically ill is the possibility of disagreement between the sick person and others as to the extent of his illness. Strauss and Glaser call this *discrepant assessments of normality*. One discrepancy is that the sick person believes he is more ill than caregivers and significant others believe him to be. In such a case, the not-really-sick individual receives the secondary gains Parsons refers to by default. More often, the sick person believes his condition is more normal than others believe it to be. In this case, they encourage the individual to withdraw and take it easy.

Most chronic illnesses have a downward trajectory that necessitates continual redefinition of normality by the sick person. The process of coming to terms with lower levels of normality is eased by the fact that symptoms and trajectories stabilize for long periods of time. Eventually, however, the chronically ill person must face the adjustment to a lower level of functioning, less normal than his previous life-style.

Moos (1977) furthers this notion by stating that chronic disease requires the development of a new equilibrium that reflects permanently altered circumstances. This involves increased dependence and new limitations on functional abilities.

The chronically ill renal dialysis patient experiences many of the sick role expectations outlined by Fox and Parsons. Though he may be maintained by mechanical intervention, he faces a downward trajectory described by Glaser and Strauss. The sick self of the dialysand is always in a state of flux as he goes in and out of periods of health, renegotiating his role as a sick person.

Other than Fox, it is interesting that most of the literature on renal dialysis patients does not apply sick role theory to patient behavior, nor does it borrow from theory on chronic illness. The dialysis patient is a contradiction: He is terminal and he is chronic, he is sick and he is not sick. The research on patient behavior has been predicated upon psychological explanation and has, consequently, not drawn upon studies outside of psychology. As a result, the body of knowledge on sick role theory is minimally considered.

Biological Influences of Behavior

There are numerous physical complications accompanying renal failure. Levine (1978) cites multiple problems: bone degeneration, skin disease, blindness, malnutrition, anemia, chronic fatigue, hepatitis, neurological complications, and dialysis dementia.

With these complications comes the speculation as to how much these affect behavior. Kemph (1966) maintains that many neuropsychiatric manifestations are probably caused by the chemical changes found in renal failure. The onset of renal failure brings about fatigue, drowsiness, and apathy. More serious uremia produces anorexia, which causes disturbances of consciousness and intellect.

Teschan (1975) suggests that behavior of renal dialysis patients should be perceived as being influenced by disordered brain function. This is caused by the dysfunction of neurochemical environment imposed by renal failure. This manifests itself in dysfunctional adaptation of the personality. Another proponent of this theory is Cummings (1970) who contends that the presence of toxins in the system causes an affect on the patient's feeling level, behavior, and interaction with staff. From clinical observations, the author claims that every dialysis candidate is experiencing at least some degree of mild organic brain dysfunction.

Some of the behavioral changes caused by biochemical imbalance are irritability, fluctuating mood, poor concentration, and mental fatigue. Neurological symptoms of insomnia, anorexia, nausea, weakness, and impotence are also reported (Foster, Cohn, and McKegney, 1973). The authors conclude that these behavioral changes and neurological symptoms give evidence to a state of dialysis-modified uremic encephalopathy.

Recent literature reflects frequent findings of a type of organic brain syndrome. This condition is given various titles and may be referred to as dementia dialytica, dialysis encephalopathy, uremic encephalopathy, and renal dementia (Menzies and Stewart, 1968; Schieber and Ziesat, 1976; Short and Durham, 1969). This syndrome is described as a progressive, irreversible, fatal psychotic organic brain syndrome. Symptoms are speech disorder (stuttering or slurring), dysparthria, dysphasia, mutism, myoclonic jerks, and final global dementia. Paranoid ideation and psychotic behavior may also appear. Most patients, according to Schieber and Ziesat (1976), die within six months of the onset of dementia dialytica. The etiology of this syndrome is not known. Hypotheses offered include a viral origin or a heavy trace metal imbalance.

These findings indicate that the effect of biochemical imbalance may range from mild, neurotic behaviors in dialysis patients to severe, psychotic brain syndrome resulting in death. Whatever the etiology of the syndrome, there is general agreement among researchers that behavioral disturbance in these patients is often linked to neurochemical causes. The differentiation between those behaviors that are neurologically induced and those that are psychologically initiated constitutes a fine line of distinction. Any comprehensive approach to provide therapeutic intervention for these patients must involve both interpretations.

Stages of Adjustment

A number of studies have outlined various stages of adjustment that have been observed in the renal dialysis patient. Reichsman and Levy (1972) report that most dialysis patients pass through three stages before adapting to dialysis. These stages are the honeymoon period, the disenchantment period, and the period of long-term adaptation. The honeymoon period is described as taking place during the first few weeks of dialysis in which the patient experiences marked physical and emotional improvement. There is general acceptance of dependency upon the machine and staff. Anxiety about one's life expectancy and ability to resume a normal life style is to be expected. Feelings of contentment diminish markedly in the disenchantment period ranging from three to twelve weeks duration. These feelings are usually preceded by the patient trying unsuccessfully to resume his old life-style. Dietary indiscretion increases during this period, which commonly leads to feelings of guilt. Displacement of anger on to the staff and family members is frequently observed. Long-term adaptation is a gradual transition in which the patient exhibits some degree of acceptance of the limitations and complications of dialysis. Long states of enchantment occur with brief episodes of depression. The patient will experience fluctuations in affect and a keen awareness of dependence on the machine. Patients continue to seek support from the staff to fulfill dependency needs.

Similar to this model, Ebra (1975) reports three loosely defined stages he observed with his patients. First, the dialysand experiences an initial reaction to the disability. Secondly, the patient goes through the actual process of adjustment. New life-styles and redefinition of previous roles are developed. Thirdly, an achievement of a successful level of rehabilitation is reached.

Due to the fact that without regular dialysis patients would die, end-stage renal failure is considered terminal. The threat of death for this patient is a constant one even though it is often denied. Kübler-Ross (1969) found that patients with terminal illness experience five stages of emotional reaction to such diagnosis: denial, anger, bargaining, depression, and acceptance. The author acknowledges that the patient can advance or recede to any of these stages throughout the illness. When one experiences a remission, he may need to rework the stages previously advanced.

Levy (1976) has suggested that these definable stages were seen more often in the previous decade when patients were taken on dialysis in an acute stage. Czaczkes and De-Nour (1978) maintain that they have never observed the honeymoon stage. Trieschmann and Sand (1971) found elevated scores of the depression scale of the MMPI on patients with terminal renal failure before initiation of dialysis. This suggests that what was thought to be a reaction to dialysis per se is expressed even before the treatment.

All the stages presented relate the emotional reactions that the chronically ill and terminally ill dialysis patient expresses when faced with chronic hemodialysis. The studies that have presented stages of emotional reactions have been conducted on small samples through clinical observations of the authors. The stages described offer guidelines to practitioners, but cannot be considered substantiated research. The following section deals with personality characteristics frequently observed in those patients who have adjusted to the dialysis regimen.

Personality Characteristics of Adjustment

Why some patients adjust to dialysis and why others do not has been a constant question of behavioralists observing this population. The characteristics that appear most frequently in the literature of the adjusted patient are: average or above average intelligence, low percentage of denial, strong family support, low anxiety, and high levels of motivation (Ebra, 1975; Levy, 1974; Sand, Livingston, and Wright, 1966). The variable of intelligence has yielded conflicting evidence. The authors above report that patients with higher IQ adjust better than those with lower IQ. Others report that there is no significant correlation between IQ and compliance with diet or rehabilitation (Cummings, 1970; Winokur, Czaczkes, and De-Nour, 1973).

Borkman (1976) maintains that there are three views in the literature relating to intelligence of renal dialysis patients. He contends that none of these views is sufficiently supported by empirical evidence. The first view is that intelligent patients adjust successfully to dialysis. The second view states that a patient's understanding of the regimen, not his intelligence, is crucial. The final stance considers intelligence as an unimportant variable. Borkman found that most health care professionals believe that intelligence has a positive influence on patient adaptation even though there is contradictory evidence relating otherwise. Patients whom staff perceive as being intelligent were found to receive different treatment than the less intelligent. Borkman claims this is a self-fulfilling prophecy engendered by staff bias.

Norton (1969) describes the "adaptive" type as that patient who has a history of success in employment and is not prone to denying the extent of his illness. Anxiety and depression are openly expressed during the early phases of dialysis.

Prolonged exposure to dialysis increases the need for social desirability (Gentry and Davis, 1972). Thus, the adapting patient experiences a need to behave in a culturally acceptable manner in order to receive sanctions from the staff. According to Brown (1963), this need poses problems for the self-reliant individual who has maintained himself as the subject center of reality previous to dialysis.

Brand and Komarita (1966) mention that those who had been experiencing renal failure for a period of time preceding dialysis shared in the decision to go on dialysis. As a result, these patients adjusted better than those who had no part in the decision. The type of patient who has not participated in the decision usually has suffered acute renal failure and was in no condition to make such a decision.

Dialysis was considered a life-saving treatment. Once over the crisis, the patient must adjust not only to dialysis but also to the fact that he is terminal.

How renal patients adapt to group life was compared to Lifton's (1967) theories regarding survivor behavior of Hiroshima victims by Foster et al. (1973). Behaviors that both populations share are immersion into death, guilt over surviving, psychic numbing, a disruption of interpersonal relationships, and unresolved grief over death of other companions sharing the same experience. The authors found that patients who did not identify with the group adapted better than those who felt part of the group. These nonparticipating group members of the dialysis unit did not identify with the sick role nor did they take on any negative group affect. These high constraint types refused to be identified with other patients, were unwilling to perform group tasks, and felt no responsibility for other patients.

Kimball (1969) addressed himself to heart transplant patients and found that adjusted patients were those who had coped successfully with previous life stresses, those who had been able to express their anxieties about possible death, and those who had multiple object relations in the past and plan to continue them in the future. He suggests these characteristics are similar to those found in the adjusted dialysand.

The literature records contradictory findings as to what the attributes are of the adjusted dialysis patient. Even though there might be general agreement as to the kinds of adjustment characteristics that have been observed, little information is available regarding which of these is necessary for survival. Definitions of adjustment are as varied as the methods used to research the personalities of the adjusted patient. These studies assume that whatever it is that makes someone adjust to dialysis, it is an internal adaptive function of the patient. Little attention is given to ecological factors of the unit or the patient–staff interactive process.

Predictive and Selective Criteria

Chronic hemodialysis began to attract the behavioral sciences very soon after implementation. With scarce resources and a demanding patient population, the early studies were concerned with predicting which personality traits promote or hinder adjustment to dialysis. Psychiatrists were asked to take part in selection of patients who would be best suited for dialysis and would not waste this life-saving resource. Even though today, anyone can receive dialysis treatment, there is still concern for knowing prospectively which patients will adjust and which will need special attention.

Fox and Swazey (1974) report that the six most frequently employed criteria used for accepting patients in the early days of dialysis were willingness to cooperate, medical suitability, absence of other disease, intelligence, likelihood of vocational rehabilitation, and absence of psychiatric disturbance. Those patients who had mental deficiency, came from unstable family environments, were indigent, and had criminal or poor employment records were usually excluded from dialysis programs. This indicated that social worth was part of the nonmedical criteria used in selection. The authors found in their survey of selection criteria of dialysis units that the standards developed by various committees often reflected their values of self-worth. Patients had to be able to relate to authority figures and exhibit no self-destructive tendencies. Presence of a responsible family member was considered a positive advantage for an applicant. Coping with stress and frustration tolerance were other psychosocial factors regarded as positive indicators for success.

In 1964, Scribner announced the criteria used by his Seattle group to determine "psychological suitability" for dialysis. Characteristics related to self-care constituted the first category. Those who exhibited a past life history of impulsive, irresponsible behavior or low intelligence were considered unfavorable. Patients with self-destructive wishes and inability to relate to authority figures were denied admission. The self-reliant, active patient who could participate in his care was the likely candidate. Potential for rehabilitation was the second category. A satisfactory life with the social support of a family, friends, and a job were the major indicators for acceptance. A poor work history, strained family relations, and low self-esteem were contraindications for dialysis. The final factor considered was the patient's ability to tolerate frequent and recurring stress caused by dialysis. Capacity to cope with the uncertainty of the future, medical complications, and crisis were necessary components of predicting the adaptive patient.

With increasing use of home dialysis and expanded resources, there has been a shift in selection criteria from social worth to psychological suitability (Fox and Swazey, 1974). Rarely does a present day dialysis unit refuse treatment to anyone strictly on nonmedical grounds. Abram (1974) relates that people are no longer excluded for psychiatric reasons. The role of the psychiatrist has changed from being a selector to a therapist working with the patient, family, and staff toward adjustment to dialysis.

De-Nour and Czaczkes (1976) share the same view. They believe that even though the circumstances have changed, there is a fundamental need for rehabilitation professionals to understand and predict the emotional response of the dialysand before treatment begins. This allows for preventative intervention in the early stages of adjustment. In a study determining the influence certain personality factors have on adjustment to chronic hemodialysis, the authors confirmed the assumption that it is possible to predict major aspects of adjustment. The major aspects of adjustment are defined as compliance with the diet, rehabilitation, and psychological condition. Depression, suicidal tendencies, anxiety, and psychotic complications were all indicators of the psychological condition. Staff had a slight tendency to overestimate the patient's adjustment potential. De-Nour and Czaczkes conclude that understanding specific personality traits that cause specific maladjustment provides a rational basis for focus-oriented psychotherapeutic intervention.

Borkman (1976) finds it "appalling" that health professionals in chronic hemodialysis still use nonmedical criteria to predict adjustment of beginning dialysis patients. The author maintains as does Moore (1976) that there have been no definitive studies that identify emotional problems that are absolutely contrary to effective treatment.

Considerable rethinking of the psychological practice of predicting those personalities that will adjust to dialysis has been evidenced in recent years. Most of the findings were developed in the early period of dialysis when selection was necessary. No studies, however, employed rigorous research; small samples, subjective interviews, and staff observations were the methodologies of such studies. Despite the inconclusive findings and lack of validity of predictive studies, there is evidence that the nonmedical criteria generated by these studies are still assumed to be true among dialysis caregivers.

Psychiatric Complications: The Patient

Emotional Disturbance

Life-extending treatment for end-stage renal disease includes a wide spectrum of patients that bring with them serious emotional problems (Moore, 1976). There are only a few patients who come into dialysis units in a state of mental health that allows them to adapt easily to chronic stress of renal failure. Psychiatric morbidity must be expected in this population as the stress of chronic hemodialysis can be most severe.

The frequency of emotional disturbance of dialysis patients is widely reported. Brown (1963) states that any evidence of emotional instability, overt or latent, should be considered a contraindication for chronic hemodialysis. Levine (1978) relates that the dialysis patient is less likely to die but more likely to suffer psychological damage from the long-term therapy. Despite psychological problems of the treatment, Cummings (1970) posits that these patients should not be treated for psychopathology. They are not to be considered a behavior deviancy group. He contends that it is only normal to react to these stresses that appear abnormal to an outsider.

Gelfman and Wilson (1972) share the same view. They report that the appearance of irrational behavior is actually an adaptive mechanism allowing the patient time to bring a sense of order to his life. Some of the emotional reactions they found in their patient population were passive styles of coping, negative perception of self, regressive patterns of cathective energy, withdrawal, low interest in goal-related activities, declined interested in interpersonal relationships, and a greatly reduced readiness to cope with challenging problems.

Much of what Gelfman and Wilson found is verified by patient interviews reported by other researchers (Wertzel, Vollrath, Ritz and Fesner, 1977). These patients classified themselves as being less able and less willing to communicate with others. Isolated and mistrusting, the patients felt trapped. While they perceived the dialysis environment as hostile and dangerous, they still desired better communication with the staff.

De-Nour and Czaczkes (1976) found increased aggression was evident in all the patients they treated. Aggression was greater for those for whom dependency and loss of control were less acceptable. This type of patient was likely to act-out by abusing the diet, by introjecting their aggressive feelings resulting in depression, or by projecting the aggression through psychotic behavior.

Feelings of hopelessness, anger, and anxiety are common reactions of the novice dialysis patient (Reischman and Levy, 1972). Anger is usually expressed later in the therapy; it is, however, often repressed when the patient feels staff has the power to terminate treatment. Abram (1972) points out that hopelessness towards the future is related to loss of self-image, freedom, mobility, and body functions. Dependence is used as a method to withdraw from the challenges of entering the work world which is threatening to the chronically ill patient. Nonadherence to the diet regimen is seen by Abram as a form of denial, independent acting-out, or as indirect self-destruction.

In 1968, Engel introduced the giving up–given up complex. This complex has the following five characteristics: a feeling of giving up experienced as hopelessness, a depreciated self-image, loss of gratification from personal relationships, a feeling of disruption in the sense of continuity between past, present, and future, and recurrence of memories of earlier periods of giving up. This psychological state often precedes the onset of illness. Engel considers this condition a contributing factor in altering the patient's capability to deal with concurrent pathogenic processes.

DEPRESSION. Depression is the most frequent psychiatric complication of dialysis (Anger, 1975; Hampers, Shupak, Lowrie and Lazarus, 1973). Depression is cyclic and is manifested in feelings of hopelessness and helplessness.

Crammond, Knight, and Lawrence (1967) claim that depression is due to the patient's reaction to being terminally ill. Wright (1966) states that depression occurs when the defense mechanism of denial has failed. Abram (1974) believes that the most prevalent reason for depression is that the patient experiences damaged self-esteem. The sense of being chronically ill contributes to depressive affect. Even the successful patient, according to Moore (1976), is likely to be neurotically depressed.

Reischman and Levy (1972) found that all the patients they had studied were significantly depressed before dialysis. Depressive feelings preceded symptoms of uremia in 40 percent of the patients. All of these patients had experienced a major loss before the onset of any physical symptoms. The affects they report are sadness, helplessness, feelings of abandonment, and inability to cope.

Many clinical studies have been conducted on small populations of no more than twenty-five patients. High frequency of depression is often reported. Gonzalez, Pabico, Brown, Maher, and Schreiner (1963) observed severe depression in half the patients studied; Shea, Bogden, Freeman, and Schreiner (1965) found nearly 60 percent of their patients were severely depressed. Other studies found less frequency of depression; Foster, Cohn, and McKegney (1973) reported less than 50 percent of their patients were depressed while Crammond, Knight, and Lawrence (1967) found less than a quarter of their sample in a depressed state.

Czaczkes and De-Nour (1978) describe an increase in reported depression of dialysis patients during recent years. The authors suggest that patients who are soon to be transplanted perceive dialysis as temporary and as a result are less prone to develop depression. The transplant is their hope and escape.

There is disagreement in the literature as to when depression occurs. Anger (1975) and Hampers et al. (1973) relate that depression follows soon after dialysis. Czaczkes and De-Nour contend that when the patients are first admitted to dialysis they are in poor physical condition. At this stage, Wise (1974) states that the depression is often a mixture of organic and functional etiology. Within a few weeks of dialysis treatment, there is general improvement of health and the depression is reduced. Daly (1969), in a paper presented to the First International Congress on Nephrology, reported that dialysis patients experience a mourning process as a reaction to their multiple losses. Often this becomes expressed via an "anniversary reaction" on or near the anniversary of beginning the treatment. The author cites a number of studies on depression of dialysis patients but contends that claims are often made without good evidence, and hypotheses are rarely put to the test. By using the Beck Depression Inventory (1961), the author measured depression in eighteen patients undergoing maintenance hemodialysis. Using the criteria established for general medical patients, he scored 72 percent in the moderately depressed range. Fatigability and work inhibition were reported but considered as complications of the treatment. Close to 100 percent of the patients report irritability, which Daly claims is an almost universal characteristic of this population. Loss of libido is also highly reported. The author concludes that a large proportion of dialysis patients have a depressed mood that requires considerable efforts for prevention and treatment. Rigorously defined depressive disorder was found in 22 percent of home hemodialysis patients in a study conducted by Lowry (1979) for a sample of fifty-eight patients. By using the *Diagnostic and Statistical Manual of Mental Disorders: Third Edition* (DSM-III) for diagnosing depression, Lowry found that a majority of the patients reported loss of interest or pleasure in usual activities, fatigability, and diminished ability to think or concentrate. Irritability and social withdrawal were reported for 33 percent of the patients.

The author maintains that renal failure can produce a global physical depression that can be difficult to differentiate from a depressive affect. Lowry suggests, however, that as the use of dialysis techniques to correct the organic imbalance of renal failure advances, it can be challenged that such psychological changes may be assumed to have a purely organic basis.

Today, the patient may experience predialysis depression that continues on a downward trajectory once on dialysis. With increased dialysis populations and the shortage of organs, the hope for transplants for many is unattainable; they must accept the fact that for them dialysis is a permanent condition, which becomes a contributing factor of depression.

DEPENDENCY VS. INDEPENDENCY CONFLICTS. The patient on intermittent dialysis is faced with severe regressive tendencies and conflicts with regard to independent needs versus dependent needs. He is dependent on the machine and personnel for his survival but he is expected to be independent while off the machine living a normal life.

Attitudes and conflicts of dependency commonly lead to patient management problems (Menzies and Stewart, 1968). The patient rarely feels well and finds it difficult to cope with the stress of dialysis. It is common belief among health care professionals that the major index of rehabilitation is the patient remaining or becoming gainfully employed. This expectation of independence increases this conflict in the patient.

Anger (1975) claims that the machine takes on a mother-child relationship to the patient. It is life-giving. The patient soon learns that he must depend upon the machine for his life but he also receives conflicting messages. The staff expects him to be independent but the staff also expects the patient to depend on them for medical care and advice. Since the patient is dependent on the staff, Abram (1974) observes that many patients will deny the extent of their illness. The patient feels vulnerable to staff retaliation in his weakened condition and finds it adaptive to deny the conflict.

The dependency vs. independency conflict is especially serious for the adolescent patient (Poznanski, Miller, Salguero, and Kelsh, 1978). The need for dependency caused by chronic illness interferes with the adolescent developmental task of autonomy. Families become too involved in the child's life, usually discouraging independent behavior. Body image changes cause particular embarrassment for this group. As a result, the younger dialysand restricts his social relationships and remains dependent on adults.

Norton (1969) interviewed dialysis patients asking them to rank ten items that were of most concern to them. Items that referred to dependency and loss of control were highest. Fear of life scored mid-range and fear of death ranked low.

Most of the studies on dependency vs. independency have shared the view that a machine-dependent life is very stressful to the patient. Over the years, however, the approach to this problem has been changing. Observations are recorded that verify patients who enjoy the dependency on dialysis (De-Nour and Czaczkes, 1976; Levy, 1976; Reichsman and Levy, 1972). For these patients, the secondary sick gains become a satisfactory role fulfilling dependency needs.

The literature on dependency vs. independency conflicts leads one to conclude that for some patients the dependency on dialysis is most stressful, for others it contributes minimal stress, and for some it is no stress at all. There is general agreement that the deciding factor on whether or not the dependency is stressful is the patient's level of dependency needs and the degree to which he accepts these needs (Czaczkes and De-Nour, 1978).

SUICIDE. There is contradictory information in the literature regarding the frequency of suicide among renal dialysis patients. The discrepancy begins with varying definitions of suicide. Abram et al. (1971) studying 3,478 dialysis patients defined suicidal patients as those who died from exsanguination, overdosage, or food and drink binges. Approximately one out of every twenty patients had committed active or passive suicide. Active suicide is defined as a direct act of taking one's life; passive suicide is seen as knowingly abusing the medical regimen in such a way as to cause death. Goldstein (1972) rejects food and drink binges as being suicidal. The author contends that the renal dialysis patient does not see his behavior as controlling or direct. As a chronically ill person, he perceives his behavior as unrelated to his condition. He adopts the perception that his locus of control is external; things happen at random, and he has little influence on them. Operating from this perceptual mode, Goldstein maintains that binges by this type of patient cannot be interpreted as suicidal.

Contrary to the Goldstein understanding of suicide, Hampers et al. (1973) share the opinion that the vast majority of dialysis suicides occur by dietary indiscretion, which is directly related to the stressful life-style of dialysis. Abram (1974) goes so far as to say that the uncooperative patient represents a variant of self-destructive behavior and can be considered a form of passive suicide.

Czaczkes and De-Nour (1978) consider three types of suicide: fatal suicide, attempted suicide, and suicide ideation. Self-inflicted damage by abuse of the diet is not treated as suicidal behavior nor is withdrawal of treatment. The suicide ideation patient is the individual who at some time or other expresses his wish and intention to terminate his life. In a study conducted by the authors they found that out of 100 patients, twenty-seven were suicidal risks. The majority of this group expressed suicidal thoughts of which two of them actually committed suicide. In a separate calculation of the mortality of the suicidal and the nonsuicidal patient, it was found that at the end of a five year period the mortality of the suicide patient was higher than the nonsuicide patient. Noncompliance with the diet was a major contributor to death of the suicidal patient. The authors suggest that the major problem of suicidal behavior of dialysis patients is not so much the active fatal suicide but the slow death caused by abuse of diet.

Suicidal thoughts are common in dialysis patients. Foster et al. (1973) reported that 43 percent of their patients had suicidal thoughts and that 19 percent of the patients attempted suicide.

Moore (1976) asserts that suicidal behavior in dialysis patients is considerably higher than in the rest of the population. It is Moore's contention that hemodialysis without the "deliverance" of a renal transplant is intolerable for most people and if transplant fails or becomes unattainable, then the suicide risk increases. Holcomb and MacDonald (1973) relate that 35 percent of their patients expressed suicidal thoughts while Shulman, Pacey, and Diewold (1978) reported that 46 percent of their patients had such thoughts. In reference to suicide and transplants, Abram et al. (1971) postulate that rejection or loss of the allograft can act as a significant factor of suicidal behavior as many patients place great emotional investment in a transplant. Chronic physical illness, stressful family relationships, and emotional disturbance prior to dialysis are causal factors of suicidal behavior in dialysis patients.

Suczek (1975) avows that unresolved dependency conflicts are causal factors in the suicidal behavior of many renal dialysis patients. Machine "bondage," loss of privacy, economic dependency, and feelings of insecurity add to dependency conflicts.

Though there are conflicting studies on the rate of active direct suicide of dialysis patients, there is general agreement that suicide ideation is common and does affect the mortality rate of such patients. Causes for suicidal behavior range from depression and transplant failure to dependency conflicts and absence of physical health.

In reviewing the four areas of psychiatric complications — emotional disturbance, depression, dependency vs. independency conflicts, and suicide — it becomes evident that statistical data are rare and definitions are varied. There is general acknowledgment that these complications are harmful and are associated with mortality. Causes for the complications are varied with as many studies supporting one view as those opposed. Most of the interpretations have viewed the problem as patient-centered followed by psychological explanations for the behavior reported. Only in the dependency vs. independency conflict is staff seen as a possible factor influencing patient behavior. Studies testing relationships between unit conditions or staff characteristics and frequency of a given psychiatric disturbance seem to be nonexistent.

DEFENSE MECHANISMS. There are a number of defense mechanisms manifested by the renal dialysis patient. Abram (1972) describes six major mechanisms: regression, denial, intellectualization, projection, displacement, and introjection.

Frequency of denial as the major defense mechanism of the renal dialysis population is strongly supported in the literature (Cummings, 1970; De-Nour and Czaczkes, 1976; Ebra, 1975; Reichsman and Levy, 1972; Wright, 1966). According to Ebra (1975), denial protects the personality from irreparable damage. It would be very unhealthy for a patient to completely face all the dimensions of his illness. Denial assists the patient in dealing with experiences on a daily basis rather than cumulatively. Wright (1966) asserts that there is a need to repress and deny the dependency conflicts of hemodialysis. The exaggeration of denial helps the patient avoid the full impact of the disease.

Crammond, Knight, and Lawrence (1967) found that patients use massive denial when they first realize that dialysis is a life-long treatment. It is common for a new dialysand to think that after a few treatments their kidney will start functioning again. This is what Short and Durham (1969) refer to as *flight into health*. They suggest that it may be necessary that these patients be allowed to maintain their capacity to deny in order to cope with their terminal state.

Hampers et al. (1973) also refer to denial as lessening anxieties. The frightened patient may withdraw from reality and assume a detached air, as if he were calmly accepting the treatment. This type of patient does not respond to confrontation. According to Ziarnik, Freeman, and Sherrard (1977), this patient should probably not be confronted with his denial. They contend that the more effective denial is in suppressing somatic complaints and depression, the longer the individual will live.

Cummings (1970) describes denial as having three features: suppression in which the patient distorts information presented him, grandiose appraisal of his situation that allows him to see himself suspended from the physical laws that affect everyone else, and withdrawal in which the patient reacts as a neutral observer of his condition. In all cases, the dialysand distorts his perception of the experience so that he can liken it to his own expectations and needs.

For this patient population, denial to a certain degree is considered a necessary coping mechanism for survival. Denial acts as a filter through which a limited amount of reality can advance up to the patient's level of consciousness. It also allows the patient enough time to develop internal resources that enable him to deal with the impending reality of chronic hemodialysis.

Stresses of Chronic Hemodialysis

In the early 1960s when chronic hemodialysis was mostly an area of experimental medicine, it was quickly realized that the procedure engendered psychological stress. Even though the technical and medical aspects have improved, there is strong evidence that emotional adjustment to dialysis is often below a desired level. It is a stressful event for everyone involved: for the patient, for the family, and for the staff (Czaczkes and De-Nour, 1978).

Strauss and Glaser (1975) present multiple daily living problems for the chronically ill: prevention of another medical crisis, constant control of the symptoms of the disease, respect of a prescribed regimen, prevention of social isolation, adjustment to the up and down trajectory of the illness, attempts at normalizing interactions with others, and socioeconomic worries. When life is contingent upon the proper following of a regimen via machinery, the personal identity of the patient usually becomes threatened by the mechanical nature of the treatment. The requirement that dialysis must be maintained for the rest of one's life confirms the terminality of the patient and reinforces the uncertainty of the future. Because a considerable amount of time is spent on dialysis, there are other consequences of the disease: boredom, decreased social skills, family strain, damaged self-esteem, and physical deterioration. Time devoted to the regimen is viewed by the patient as empty time. Few patients engage in meaningful activity during dialysis.

Cummings (1970) identifies the major pressure points of stress for the dialysis patient as toxic factors that influence behavior, economic insecurity, social role disturbance, imposed dependency, and sexual dysfunction. All of these pressure points affect the patient's interpersonal life.

Loss of control over one's environment is a source of stress upheld by Engel (1968). Of the patients studied by the author, all had experienced a sudden change in their environment about which the victim was powerless previous to the onset of illness. This sense of psychological impotence often causes lax implementation of the regimen by the patient. Rather than deal with the stress of restrictions and a controlling environment, the patient withdraws into passivity.

Another factor that influences stress with dialysis is uncertainty of the future and feelings of hopelessness (Jackle, 1974). Chance of improvement and the salvation of a transplant affect the life satisfaction of the patient. Moos and Tsu (1977) warn, however, that the possibility of new medical procedures can provoke stress in the patient by making the task of coping with loss more difficult. In this instance, the patient must prepare for the permanent loss of kidneys while maintaining hope that restoration of this function may yet be possible.

Three areas of stress—body image, threat of death, and family strain—are reviewed in separate sections due to the amount of attention they have received in the literature and the import stress has been given by most researchers.

THE STRESS OF BODY IMAGE CHANGE. The dialysis patient faces a number of alterations in his body image. Pallid color, bloating, loss of body parts and function, and a mechanized treatment regimen contribute to these alterations. Wijsenbeek and Muntz (1970) assert that attachment to the dialysis machine and concomitant flowing of blood outside the body are potent causes for disturbance of the integrity of body image. Menzies and Stewart (1968) also found patient anxiety over seeing their blood outside of themselves. Abram (1974) reports of a *Lazarus phenomenon* in which the patient, through an increasing awareness of seeing his blood coursing through the cannulae, realizes that realistically and symbolically he is returning from the dead.

A variety of reactions are reported regarding patient relationships to the dialysis machine. Fox and Swazey (1974) found three basic reactions: the patient found it intolerable to see his blood outside himself; others felt they were half robot, half man; and some saw it as a type of roulette wheel which played with their lives. All patients exhibited feelings of resentment, anger, and fear towards the machine. Apprehension over becoming dehumanized by the machine was frequently displayed.

Kemph (1967) describes patients who reported that they felt like the "living dead." It was as though they had incorporated the machine into their body image. Reichsman and Levy (1972) give further accounts of a college student undergoing chronic hemodialysis who likened the experience as like watching a Dracula movie. They report that these patients unconsciously think of themselves as not entirely human and somewhat freakish.

Cessation of urination creates another source of body-image anxiety. De-Nour (1969) relates that urinating is of great emotional importance to adults facing the loss of urination or actually having lost this function. The threat of loss or actual loss causes regression to pregenital stages of development and renewed hypercathexis of urination. Predialysis patients often deny that they will lose kidney function, that they will no longer urinate. Patients exaggerate the remains of this function, which leads to the appearance of phantom urination after the nephrectomy. Essentially, the patient reacts to this loss of urinating by mobilizing denial to a degree of classical phantom phenomena. It is common to witness urinary competition with other patients in the dialysis unit. Status is ascribed to the patient who is still able to produce urinary output, no matter how slight. Basch (1974) described phantom sensations in dialysis along with the pride transplanted patients display in being able to urinate. De-Nour suggests that urination for the normal adult symbolizes aggressiveness rather than the eroticism attached to urination during childhood. Tourkow (1974) commented on the significance the lack of urination has for men rather than women while Wijsenbeek and Munitz (1970) have described how lack of urination leads to sexual fear and impotency for men. Both studies emphasize that loss of urination causes considerable anxiety for the dialysis patient.

Though the general physical health and hormonal level is improved with dialysis, sexual function is found to deteriorate in both men and women (Czaczkes and De-Nour, 1978). The authors posit four explanations for this. First, a decrease in sexual function may be caused by organic factors as some patients become more anemic on dialysis than in the uremic stage. Neuropathy on dialysis is also reported. Secondly, patients have a tendency to glorify their past sexual abilities. It might have well been that they experienced the same sexual problems previous to dialysis but use dialysis as an excuse for their present difficulties. Thirdly, changes in marital relations may also influence sexual anxiety. The authors relate findings that spouses also become anxious about sexual relations. Changes in family roles, especially with male patients, add to frustrated sexual activity.

Finally, psychological complications contribute to sexual dysfunction. The high incidence of depression among dialysis patients influences the weakening of the sexual drive. Steele, Finklestein, and Finklestein (1976) found a strong relationship between severity of depression and severity of sexual inadequacy in patients but not in spouses.

The frequency of decreased libido among dialysis patients has been recently reported in the literature. Studies indicating that at least half the male patients sampled experienced impotency are frequent (Abram et al., 1975; Larsen, 1972; Levy, 1974; Foster et al., 1973). Larsen reports that the frequency of intercourse in women is also drastically reduced. He reports that 65 percent of the women on dialysis do not have intercourse, while others (Dubernard, Moskovtchenko, Barnay, and Cognet, 1974) report lower figures of 30 percent. According to most reports, 50 percent to 65 percent of the women have no libido at all.

There appear to be three factors that influence sexual functioning; patients can be expected to experience sexual activities if they are in very good physical condition, if the marital relationship is satisfactory, and if there is minimal depression (Czaczkes and De-Nour, 1978).

THE THREAT OF DEATH. Fear of death has often been cited as a major source of stress for the dialysand (Beard, 1969; Goldstein and Reznikoff, 1971; Sand et al., 1966). This school of thought argues that the stress of impending death is acute in hospital-based units since patients are in a group setting and witness each other's death. Anger (1975) contends that one of the greatest underlying stresses faced by the dialysis patient is his ultimate fear of death as he becomes part of two worlds: that of the living and that of the dying. The mortality rate of dialysis patients is high, thus the possibility of death is not only a threat but an actuality (De-Nour and Czaczkes, 1976). In a study by Beard (1969), all his patients described imminent fear of impending death as a constant source of emotional strain. Denial was a common defense used to suppress anxieties about dying. Kemph (1967) observed that during the pretransplant period depressive trends of the patients were directly related to the fear of death. Hampers et al. (1973) mention that whether a transplant is performed or the patient remains on dialysis, the individual must come to terms with the gravity of his illness, i.e. the likely proposition of an early death. An editorial in the *Journal of the American Medical Association* (1968) declared that the person who lives successfully with hemodialysis lives in a state of "suppressed inner turmoil for which there can never be an escape, except death."

Other studies have rejected the premise that fear of death is a major stress factor. Gelfman and Wilson (1972) argue that the fear of death is more of a factor with the patient's family and the caregivers than with the patient. Fear of death is a secondary issue to the patient. The loss of control, the strict regimen, and poor quality of life are more stressful to the patient than possible death. Some have presented the idea that the patient may be more afraid of life than death. De-Nour and Czaczkes (1976) question whether or not this may be true; perhaps these patients mobilize denial more than their counterparts who express fear of death.

The issue of the quality of life on hemodialysis is the other dimension of the fear of death. Abram (1974) postulates that the fear of death affects most cardiac patients but the fear of living affects most renal dialysis patients. Ebra (1975) surmises that the dialysand is probably equally afraid of living as he is of dying. The prospect of living under the constant threat of death, living as a disabled person, and being dependent upon a machine for life are frightening and overwhelming. For the remainder of one's life, Abram (1975) remarks, the patient must wrestle at both conscious and unconscious levels with the question, "Is life on dialysis worth living?" Neither dialysis nor transplantation is viewed by Fox (1976) as releasing the patient from this chronic way of dying. Beard (1969) sees the fear of death coupled with the fear of life as the existential dilemma of the dialysis patient.

How much the fear of death affects patient adjustment to chronic hemodialysis is debatable. The literature documents two points of view: the threat of death causes acute stress or the threat of death is minimal in comparison to the patient's fear of living. Little reference is given to recent studies of death anxiety or use of death anxiety scales being generated in thanatology. Studies on staff anxiety toward death or evaluation of the coping skills they have developed to deal with death are infrequent.

FAMILY STRESS. The reported frequency of pathological reactions in families indicates that hemodialysis is stressful for the family. Eisendrath (1969) observes that one area of concern for the medical recovery of the patient involves an understanding of the patient's relationship to his family. The interpersonal relationships within the family, according to Hampers et al. (1973), have a great impact on adjustment. The family support system influences the patient's outlook on his treatment.

This resource of support, however, is faced with adverse pressure that abates its potential strength. A number of possible sources of stress for the spouse have been suggested. Friedman, Goodwin, and Chaudhry (1970) report that the decrease in economic and financial status is a serious source of family stress. Short and Wilson (1969) also speak to economic worries that contribute to the uncertainty of the future. More severe than the economy to family relations is the stress dialysis plays upon the marital role. The continued pressures cause the spouse to become more distant to his or her partner. The dialysand is forced to become more dependent and represses feelings of guilt and aggression from this dependency. Levy (1973) notes that there is a tendency for reversal of family role, especially in the case of the male patient. The patient usually becomes less productive, which indirectly causes a reduction of income. The hemodialysis patient, who is chronically anemic, intermittently uremic, and exposed to many medical complications, is not in a position to assume previous emotional involvement with his spouse and children. This loss of affect places added stress upon family intradynamics.

In a study by Shulman et al. (1978), patients assessed as poorly adjusted were viewed by their spouse as being a severe burden while the spouses of well-adjusted patients were considered only a mild burden by their spouse. This suggests that there is a relationship between spousal perception of stress and patient adjustment. In 1976, Maurin and Schenkel studied the family unit's response to dialysis. They report finding the patient exhibiting great levels of control. There is minimal open communication among all family members with obvious omission of the children.

The stressfulness of hemodialysis for spouses is contingent upon previous levels of dependency needs (Czaczkes and De-Nour, 1978). For the dominant spouse, dialysis is not stressful while for the basically dependent spouse, dialysis will be stressful. In this case, dependency needs will be solicited from others. The frustration of dependency needs impels increased aggression that causes the spouse to cope with two kinds of stress: the frustration of his needs and his own increased aggression. This initiates an endless cycle of frustration for both patient and spouse.

The literature makes it clear that life on dialysis is most stressful. The studies give a descriptive account of the multiple sources of stress: fear of death and living, machine dependency, body image deterioration, marital strain, and loss of control. There are conflicting findings as to what stress causes what reactions or as to which is more serious. When stress is discussed, it is usually treated unilaterally rather than interactively. Each group—family, patient, and staff—are reported separately. Few studies review what affect a particular stress has on all components of the dialysand's world.

The usual methods of data gathering have been observations on small groups by a staff psychiatrist. Sources of the stress are speculated, few being substantiated by research. The literature lacks a differentiation between defining those stresses that are inherent in the treatment and those that could be modified.

References

Abram, H.S.: The psychology of chronic illness. *Journal of Chronic Disease*, 25:659-664, 1972.

Abram, H.S.: Psychiatric reflections on adaptation to repetitive dialysis. *Kidney International*, 6:67-72, 1974.

Abram, H.S., Hester, L.R., Sheridan, W.F., and Epstein, G.M.: Sexual functioning with chronic renal failure. *Journal of Nervous and Mental Disease*, 160:220-233, 1975.

Abram, H.S., Moore, G.L., and Westervelt, F.B.: Suicidal behavior in chronic dialysis patients. *American Journal of Psychiatry*, 127:1119-1204, 1971.

Anger, D.: The Psychologic Stress of Chronic Renal Failure and Long-term Hemodialysis. *Nursing Clinics of North America*, 10:449-460, 1975.

Basch, S.: Adaptation to dialysis and body image. *Proceedings of the 5th International Congress of Nephrology*, 3:211-220, 1974.

Beard, B.H.: Fear of death and fear of life—the dilemma in chronic renal failure, hemodialysis, and kidney transplantation. *Archives of General Psychiatry*, 21:373-380, 1969.

Beck, A.T., Ward, C.H., Mendelson, M., Mock, J., and Erbaugh, J.: An inventory for measuring depression. *Archives of General Psychiatry*, 4:53-63, 1961.

Borkman, T.S.: Hemodialysis compliance: The relationship of staff estimates of patient's intelligence and understanding to compliance. *Social Science and Medicine*, 10:385-393, 1976.

Brand, L., and Komarita, N.I.: Adapting to long-term hemodialysis. *American Journal of Nursing*, 66:1778-1781, 1966.

Brown, E.L.: Meeting patients' psychosocial needs in the general hospital. *The*

Annals of the American Academy of Political and Social Sciences, 346:118-123, 1963.

Crammond, W.A., Knight, P.R., and Lawrence, J.R.: The psychiatric contribution to a renal unit undertaking chronic hemodialysis and renal homotransplantation. *British Journal of Psychiatry,* 113:1201-1212, 1967.

Cummings, J.W.: Hemodialysis—Feelings, facts, and fantasies. *American Journal of Nursing,* 70:70-76, 1970.

Czaczkes, J.W., and De-Nour, A.K.: *Chronic Hemodialysis as a Way of Life.* New York, Brunner Mazel Publishers, 1978.

Daly, R.J.: Psychiatric aspects of maintenance hemodialysis. *Proceedings of the IVth International Congress on Nephrology,* 3:121-130, 1969.

De-Nour, A.K.: Some notes on the psychological significance of urination. *Journal of Nervous and Mental Disease,* 148:615-618, 1969.

De-Nour, A.K., and Czaczkes, J.W.: The influence of patient's personality on adjustment to chronic dialysis. *Journal of Nervous and Mental Disease,* 162:323-333, 1976.

Dubernard, C., Moskovtchenko, J.F., Barnay, C., and Cognet, M.: Approche psychologique de la genitalite et de la sexualite chez la femme en hemodialyse. *Journal d'Urologie et Nephrologie,* 4-5:377-379, 1974.

Ebra, G.: Our experience in end-stage renal disease. In Goodman, A. (Ed.): *New Dimensions of Health Care in End-stage Renal Disease.* Washington, D.C., U.S. Department of Health, Education and Welfare, 1975.

Editorial: On borrowed time. *Journal of the American Medical Association,* 5:195, 1968.

Eisendrath, R.M.: The role of grief and fear in death of kidney patients. *American Journal of Psychiatry,* 126:381-387, 1969.

Engel, G.L.: A life setting conducive to illness—the giving up-given up complex. *Annals of Internal Medicine,* 69:293-300, 1968.

Foster, G.F., Cohn, G.L., and McKegney, F.P.: Psychobiologic factors and individual survival on chronic renal hemodialysis—A two year follow-up: Part I. *Psychosomatic Medicine,* 35:64-71, 1973.

Fox, R.C.: *Experiment Perilous.* Glencoe, Illinois, The Free Press, 1959.

Fox, R.C.: Long-term dialysis programs: New selection criteria, new problems. *Hastings Center Report,* 3:8-13, 1976.

Fox, R.C., and Swazey, J.P.: *The Courage to Fail: A Social View of Organ Transplants and Dialysis.* Chicago, the University of Chicago Press, 1974.

Friedman, E.A., Goodwin, N.J., and Chaudhry, L.: Psychosocial adjustment of family maintenance hemodialysis: II. *New York State Journal of Medicine,* 70:767, 1970.

Gelfman, M. and Wilson, E.J.: Emotional reactions in a renal unit. *Comprehensive Psychiatry,* 13:283-290, 1972.

Gentry, W.D., and Davis, G.C.: Cross-sectional analysis of psychological adaptation to chronic hemodialysis. *Journal of Chronic Diseases,* 25:545-555, 1972.

Goldstein, A.M.: The subjective experience of denial in an objective investigation of chronically ill patients. *Psychosomatics,* 13:20-23, 1972.

Goldstein, A.M., and Reznikoff, M.: Suicide in chronic hemodialysis patients from an external locus of control framework. *American Journal of Psychiatry,* 127:1204-1207, 1971.

Gonzalez, F.M., Pabico, R.C., Brown, W.H., Maher, J.F., and Schreiner, G.E.: Further experience with the use of routine intermittent hemodialysis in chronic renal failure. *Transactions American Society for Artificial Internal Organs, 15*:347, 1969.

Hampers, C., Schupak, E., Lowrie, E., and Lazarus, J.M.: *Long-term Hemodialysis: The Management of the Patient with Chronic Renal Failure (2nd edition)*. New York, Grune and Stratton, 1973.

Holcomb, J.L., and MacDonald, R.W.: Social functioning of artificial kidney patients. *Social Science and Medicine, 7*:109-119, 1973.

Jackle, M.J.: Life satisfaction and kidney dialysis. *Nursing Forum, 13*:360-370, 1974.

Kemph, J.P.: Psychotherapy with patients receiving kidney transplants. *American Journal of Psychiatry, 5*:124-128, 1966.

Kimball, C.P.: Psychological responses to the experiences of open heart surgery. *American Journal of Psychiatry, 126*:348-359, 1969.

Kübler-Ross, E.: *On Death and Dying*. New York, Macmillan Co., 1969.

Larsen, N.A.: Sexual problems of patients on renal dialysis treatment and after renal transplantation. *Proceedings. European Dialysis and Transplant Association, 9*:271, 1972.

Levine, C.: Dialysis or transplant: Values and choices. *Hastings Center Report, 8*:8-10, 1978.

Levy, N.B.: The psychology and care of the maintenance hemodialysis patient. *Heart and Lung, 2*:400-405, 1973.

Levy, N.B. (Ed.): *Living or Dying — Adaptation to Hemodialysis*. Springfield, Illinois, Charles C Thomas, 1974.

Levy, N.B.: Coping with maintenance hemodialysis: Psychological considerations in the care of patients. In Massry, S.G., and Sellers, A.L. (Eds.): *Clinical Aspects of Uremia and Hemodialysis*, Springfield, Illinois, Charles C Thomas, 1976.

Lifton, R.J.: *Death in Life: Survivors of Hiroshima*. New York, Random House, 1967.

Lowry, M.R.: Frequency of depressive disorders in patients entering home dialysis. *Journal of Nervous and Mental Disease, 167*:199-203, 1979.

Maurin, J., and Schenkel, J.: A study of the family unit's response to hemodialysis. *Journal of Psychosomatic Research, 20*:163, 1976.

Menzies, I.C., and Stewart, W.K.: Psychiatric observations on patients receiving regular dialysis treatments. *British Medical Journal, 1*:544-547, 1968.

Moore, G.L.: Psychiatric aspects of chronic renal disease. *Postgraduate Medicine, 60*:140-146, 1976.

Moos, R.H. (Ed.): *Coping with Physical Illness*. New York, Plenum Medical Books, 1977.

Moos, R.H., and Tsu, V.D.: The crisis of physical illness: An overview. In Moos, R.H. (Ed.): *Coping with Physical Illness*. New York, Plenum Medical Books, 1977.

Norton, C.E.: Attitudes towards living and dying in patients on chronic hemodialysis. *Annals of the New York Academy of Science, 164*:720, 1969.

Parsons, T.: *The Social System*. Glencoe, Illinois, The Free Press, 1951.

Poznanski, E.O., Miller, E., Salguero, C., and Kelsh, R.: Quality of life for long-term survivors of end-stage renal disease. *Journal of American Medical Association,*

239:2343-2347, 1978.
Reichsman, R., and Levy, N.B.: Problems in adaptation to maintenance hemodialysis. *Archives of Internal Medicine, 130*:859-865, 1972.
Sand, P., Livingston, G., and Wright, R.G.: Psychological assessment of candidates for hemodialysis program. *Annals of Internal Medicine, 64*:602, 1966.
Scheiber, S.C., and Ziesat, H.: Dementia Dialytica—A new psychotic organic brain syndrome. *Comprehensive Psychiatry, 17*:781-785, 1976.
Scribner, B.H.: Ethical problems of using artificial organs to sustain life. *Transactions of the American Society for Artificial Internal Organs, 10*:209-212, 1964.
Shea, E.J., Bogan, D.F., Freeman, R.B., and Schriner, G.: Hemodialysis for chronic renal failure IV—Psychological considerations. *Annals of Internal Medicine, 62*:558, 1965.
Short, M.J., and Wilson, W.P.: Roles of denial in chronic hemodialysis. *Archives of General Psychiatry, 20*:433-447, 1969.
Shulman, R., Pacey, I., and Diewold, P.: The quality of life on home dialysis. In Czaczkes, J.W., and De-Nour, A.K. (Eds.): *Chronic Hemodialysis as a Way of Life*. New York, Brunner Mazel, 1978.
Steele, T.E., Finklestein, F.O., and Finklestein, S.H.: Hemodialysis patients and spouses—Marital discord, sexual problems, and depression. *Journal of Nervous and Mental Disease, 162*:225, 1976.
Strauss, A., and Glaser, B.: *Chronic Illness and the Quality of Life*. St. Louis, C.V. Mosby Company, 1975.
Suczek, B.: Chronic renal failure and the problem of funding. In Strauss, A., and Glaser, B. (Eds.): *Chronic Illness and the Quality of Life*. St. Louis, C.V. Mosby Company, 1975.
Teschan, P.E.: The psychological effects of renal failure. In Goodman, A. (Ed.): *New Dimensions of Health Care in End-stage Renal Disease*. Washington, D.C., U.S. Department of Health, Education and Welfare, 1975.
Tourkow, L.P.: Psychic consequences of loss and replacement of body parts. *Journal of the American Psychoanalytic Association, 22*:170, 1974.
Trieschmann, R.B., and Sand, P.: WAIS and MMPI correlates of increasing renal failure in adult medical patients. *Psychological Reports, 29*:1251, 1971.
Wertzel, H., Vollrath, P., Ritz, E., and Ferner, E.: Analysis of patient-nurse interaction in hemodialysis units. *Journal of Psychosomatic Research, 21*:259-266, 1977.
Wijsenbeek, H., and Munitz, H.: Group treatment in a hemodialysis center. *Psychitria Neurologia, Neurochirurgia, 73*:213, 1970.
Winokur, M.Z., Czaczkes, J.W., and De-Nour, A.K.: Intelligence and adjustment to chronic hemodialysis. *Journal of Psychosomatic Research, 17*:29-34, 1973.
Wise, T.N.: The pitfalls of diagnosing depression in chronic renal failure. *Psychosomatics, 15*:83, 1974.
Wright, K.G.: Psychological stress during hemodialysis for chronic renal failure. *Annals of Internal Medicine, 64*:607-610, 1966.
Ziarnik, J.P., Freeman, C.W., and Sherrard, D.R.: Psychological correlates of survival on renal dialysis. *Journal of Nervous and Mental Disease, 164*:210-213, 1977.

III.
THE PEDIATRIC UROLOGY PATIENT

Chapter 21

EMOTIONAL EFFECTS OF CHRONIC UROLOGIC ILLNESS ON CHILDREN

Leah Beck

IT is important to recognize the remarkable ability of most children who have lived with chronic illness and a grave prognosis to accept and grow under the shadow of very threatening and often debilitating illness. In dealing with the darker side, we often need an overall view to remind us of the other aspects. This does not infer that because children and their families are basically emotionally healthy that they are not entitled to maximum relief of suffering. They are entitled to as much relief as those who cope less successfully. Our job is to minimize suffering by direct interaction either on a one-to-one basis or in child, family, and parent groups, or with medical, nursing, and dietary staff. The aim is to help staff deal with their own personal emotions and to help them work with children and families who do and do not exhibit maladaptive patterns. The goal is to facilitate functioning and growth in the child patient regardless of ultimate outcome.

What are the emotional effects of chronic urologic illness on children? There is no simple answer; much depends on the age, familial cluster, intelligence and personality of the child, length of the chronicity, number of procedures performed, and even the school that the child attends and the community in which he lives.

Since intermittent hospitalization plays a prominent role in chronicity, it is appropriate to discuss how children at various developmental stages view hospitalization. What are their most prominent anxieties? The presenting anxiety at each hospitalization is usually age related, except for acute situations. Early in infancy until about six months of age, the infant himself does not directly feel the anxiety. It is transmitted to him or her by the mother, father, or other caregivers who are aware of the implications. The communication is by sensory reception, touch, and feel; by the way the baby is held and fed. The anxiety resides with the parents because they have the apparatus to interpret the information, and from that point of view, they need support that can then transmit its results to the infant.

From about six months to three years of age, the principal anxiety is separation anxiety. No matter how painful or difficult a procedure the child may endure, his biggest fear is being motherless. His memory is not sufficiently developed to recall a procedure for any length of time. His better recall is being away from mother. Separation anxiety reaches its peak at eighteen months and gradually decreases until age three. It actually never completely leaves, even in adulthood.

However, at age three, a new and more pressing anxiety emerges as the other one becomes less important and threatening. The new anxiety is fear of mutilation. Until three years of age, the child does not have a good concept of body image. He is just beginning to develop this at twenty months of age. At about two and one-half years old, he will retain constancy of image up to adolescence. He will get taller, broader, fatter, or thinner, but he or she will still look like the same child. Along with this awareness, he begins to realize how little and vulnerable he is. Another area of growth is the emerging sense of identity, with intense body interest and curiosity. The big fear is about what is going to be done to that body. This is the beginning of fear of punishment and of any changes to the body image. To the physically normal child as well as to the chronically ill, it is the BandAid® age. A child can have an enormous surgical procedure and call the doctor's attention to a slight cut or bruise, and it is all cured by a BandAid.

Following this stage, but certainly not obliterating the others, the most verbalized fear from ages five to seven is death. Although the finite, irreversible concept of death is certainly beyond the psyche of most children of this age, they think this is the worst thing that can happen to them. It is the just punishment and retaliation for all unacceptable wishes and thoughts at that age or any other. Again, the earlier fears have not completely gone away. They simply occupy less prominent places in the conscious mind.

From seven to ten or eleven, the child's fears seem to be centered around loss of material objects (siblings, pets, games) and fear of internal as well as external mutilation. By that age, the child has realized that he has insides and he is fearful of how they may be rearranged.

At almost ten or eleven, and particularly with boys, there is still another plague, the fear of disgrace. Will he break down and cry like a baby or be brave like a man even if he isn't one yet? Our culture may be unfair to women later, but is particularly unfair to boys when they are growing up. I am talking about our expectation that little boys do not show emotions, and most particularly do not cry.

The same child with the same chronic illness may have different fears at different stages in his life. As he gets older, they relate to specific kinds of disability. Along with the fears, there is also the hope (and this should never be overlooked) of things being better. However, sometimes the hope can far surpass the possibilities, and the child does need help to bring it into a realistic focus. Often the chronically and possibly fatally ill child nurses the fantasy that when he grows up "everything will be all right." When this does not occur, the teenager runs the danger of becoming completely negative and rebellious at the tyranny of his chronic medical regime. As we know, there is a natural rebelliousness at adolescence to which children are entitled. However, it can interfere with the medical routine necessary to maintain optimum health.

Understanding the fears and hopes of patient and family can help to care for them. In spite of the generalizations implied above, each child is an individual, each family constellation different, and each case needs individual appraisal to determine strengths and weaknesses.

We must also understand the coping devices that each child and family has developed as reactions to chronic and acute illness. The human being has just so many defenses in his repertoire, and he brings to this situation, as to any other anxiety-provoking situation, all that he has to offer. The most universal defense is repression of affect (emotions, anxiety, and anger), and the other common one is denial. If these defenses are not overdone and serve well, they can help families through ordeals. When they are unrealistic and interfere, they must be dealt with. Additional defenses are regression, projection, and displacement, and these can create management problems unless understood.

Who then are the urologic patients with chronic illness who are in danger of dying? In the past fifteen years, there has been a remarkable shift. Although in the late 1960s or early 1970s, we would occasionally come across a child dying of chronic renal disease or Wilm's tumor, we have rarely seen them since the active use of dialysis and transplant services. What we do see are more children and adults who have to face chronic urinary tract and/or renal disease.

One of the more unusual congenital diseases of the urinary tract that we see is exstrophy of the bladder, usually with epispadias. Occasionally, we see those more unfortunate children who suffer from a combination of exstrophy with imperforate anus. Our urology service (at Babies Hospital, Columbia-Presbyterian Medical Center, New York City) has organized an exstrophy support team that includes a big brother–big sister service. The team consists of the urologist, psychiatrist, pediatrician, social worker, nurse, stoma specialist, and an additional person who acts as a coordinator and who explores the field for better collecting devices.

As part of this support effort, I arranged a session with follow-up interview for twenty-six adults (ages 17 to 24) who have lived with this condition all their lives. Some had been diverted and some had not. With one exception, they were all functioning well, educationally, vocationally, and sexually. Of those who had not been diverted, three girls and one boy developed continence in their late teens. The chief anxiety of the members of this group is, first, for continence; and then it is for sexual performance and being acceptable to the opposite sex. With the support team, much has been done to alleviate the suffering that these individuals undergo as well as to improve the quality of their lives.

Procedures for improving the quality of life for the above group and for children with other chronic urologic disorders are being further developed. One procedure is intermittent self-catheterizing for children with neurogenic bladders. It is amazing how these children and their mothers can adeptly perform this task once they have been shown proper techniques. It is a great aid in teaching the child means of coping and in allowing a living situation where there is no interference with daily routine and where the child is as much like his peers as possible.

Another new procedure for the diverted child is undiversion. It is emotionally preferable under any circumstances but especially if the child is to go on to the nephrology service. So far there have been about ten undiversions performed. The reactions have all been positive once the patient is over the immediate postoperative reactions. In fact, the reactions have been euphoric either on the part of the child or his family. Following the euphoria when reality sets in and as often happens when toilet training is initiated, there is a simmering down. But the mood is better than before, and the self-esteem is markedly improved. If there has been depression, it is lifted. If there was no overt depression, there is a feeling of improved well-being for the family as well as the child. Ultimately, improved functioning and better socialization can lead to improvements in basic personality.

Because we have gained new steps in the care of the chronic urologic child patient, i.e. dialysis and transplant, we do not often see death in child patients. We do not prepare children for dying when we expect them to live. However, we do work with them and their families to accept the realities of life, even those lives that will be shortened. Children are encouraged to work to the optimum of their capacities, and parents are encouraged to give up their controls and to allow the growing child to perform age appropriate tasks and duties. The children are not spared from the prognosis if it is grave. Their moods are understood, and they are not given false hope. But, if realistic, hope is given, along with assurance that the patient will not be alone. Regardless of prognosis, we try to help the families and children maintain the best quality of life.

The dying child must gradually relinquish his tasks, and caregivers must take over. However, even as they are taking over more and more, they must give more and more love. The families of the dying child need support because as they are premourning their child and moving away, they must, at the same time, move closer and be more loving. This is a very paradoxical task and a difficult feat to accomplish. If successfully accomplished, it leaves parents with a minimum of guilt and a maximum of fond memories.

Chapter 22

THE ROLE OF SOCIAL WORK IN THE CARE OF THE SERIOUSLY ILL CHILD UROLOGY PATIENT

ESTHER BRAUN

THE impact of a serious urological disease on a child and his family requires an interdisciplinary approach to caregiving in order to ensure comprehensive, consistent, and individualized care. Considered in this chapter are the psychological impact of serious urological illness on child and family and the role of social work in alleviating undue stress and attaining realizable goals.

Social work has a unique responsibility in health care as a result of its knowledge of human behavior, the socioeconomic and cultural factors affecting individuals, and the interlocking relationship of all of these, particularly during the period of crisis in illness. While the social worker has a major responsibility for the psychological care of the patient, nothing less than a milieu approach can provide the quality and range of services needed when a child presents with a serious urological disease or disorder. What is required is an environment that is nutritive and supportive physically and emotionally for the child, so that his full recuperative powers can be mobilized. This can be achieved only through the cooperative effort of concerned professionals with clearly defined, child-centered objectives that involve the family in planning to the fullest extent possible.

The family's response to the crisis of major illness and the coping mechanisms called into play are of crucial importance. Parental guilt, anger, depression, and denial need to be dealt with, and in the case of the critically or terminally ill child, they need to be channeled into normal grief. No two cases are the same and printed instructions cannot be applied. However, we can try to extract some theoretical guidelines from our own experience and the experience of others working with ill children.

As a result of significant advances in the field of urology in recent years, the prognosis for many serious urological conditions is much better. Some conditions which, in the past, had spelled early death are now treatable and have been transferred into the category of chronic disease. As such, they may nevertheless require multiple surgeries and prolonged treatment to which child and family must adjust. Among the grave medical conditions seen on the Pediatric Genitourinary (G.U.) Service are Wilm's tumor; kidney failure; and end-stage renal disease (often leading to dialysis and transplant); birth defects, such as exstrophy of the bladder and spina bifida; and urological complications secondary to other serious illnesses.

With the diagnosis of Wilm's tumor, parents are suddenly faced with the fact of their child's malignant condition, which necessitates immediate major surgery. The child, who is usually under six years of age, is admitted to the hospital under crisis conditions at a time in his development when illness is viewed as punishment for being "bad" and separation from mother is almost intolerable. Siblings are hastily deposited with relatives or friends, aware that a calamity has occurred, and feeling anxious and left out. Crisis intervention by the social worker as soon as the condition is diagnosed can help maintain family stability, so important at this time. Surgery is followed, usually, by regular courses of chemotherapy extending over a period of years. There is continuing anxiety about possible recurrence. The child must endure both the acute stage of the disease as well as the long-term follow-up treatment. Chemotherapy, as we know, is accompanied by disfiguring hair loss and malaise, causing the child discomfort and interrupting his normal activities.

In end-stage renal failure, the disease has usually been preceded by years of treatment. As McCollum (1975, p. v) has expressed, "Parents of an ill or disabled child may find themselves treading a tightrope between hope and despair, perhaps for many years. Their standard and style of living may be affected significantly; every relationship within the family may be influenced." Treatment has usually been geared, over the long term, to staving off or at least slowing down the process of deterioration of kidney function. This may have involved multiple surgical procedures and a variety of medical regimens, and the child may have had a urinary diversion which requires his wearing a urinary collecting device similar to a colostomy bag.

Dialysis and kidney transplant are often not regarded as realistic prospects by family or patient until they become imminent. The reality of life dependent on a machine must then be faced. Often a nephrectomy has been performed prior to dialysis, symbolizing that there can now be no turning back. Added stresses are the issues of possible kidney donors, the disruption of normal activity due to long hours on the dialysis machine, and severe dietary restrictions. Of course, the ever-present questions arise: "When will a kidney become available?" and "Will it work?" At each stage there is the pervasive fear of death itself, in a sense an anachronism in childhood and a reality from which we all tend to recoil.

Transplantation is sometimes seen as the magic cure so fervently prayed for, but the prayers tend to ignore the qualifying and contingency aspects of a newly transplanted kidney. Being alive but moon-faced and funny-looking from steroid therapy and other immunosuppressives can be difficult to cope with for the young child as well as for the adolescent anxious to be accepted by peers.

Birth defects such as exstrophy of the bladder, various kidney anomalies, and spina bifida all present life-long management and treatment problems. The parents must come to terms with having an "imperfect" child, then with the realities of medical problems and the long-term treatment plan. It is important that support and information be made quickly available to these parents. An Exstrophy Support team, consisting of urologist, pediatrician, child-psychiatrist, nurse, and social worker, should provide these services on a continuing basis.

For the child, there begins a life-long struggle to "make it" in the so-called normal world. Facing surgeries and hospitalizations; coping with bags and urinary devices that may leak embarrassingly; feeling like a freak; dealing with social problems, body image concerns, and scapegoating both within and outside the family are all realities he may have to handle as well as his own rage and its counterpart, depression, when he asks, "Why me?"

We may tend to forget that these struggles have their ego-building aspects as well, and we should try to capitalize on that possibility. We learn from Crisis Theory that with the mastery of each new task or stressful event there is attendant strengthening of coping capacities. From a long-term follow-up of exstrophy patients (much longer than was previously possible), we noted that as a group they tend to be high achievers and are represented in many fields of endeavor. Apparently, most have been able to surmount what may surely be one of the most devastating of handicapping conditions.

Gravely ill children from other services frequently present G.U. complications requiring palliative or other measures from the urologists. While these may not be lifesaving, they are still important to reduce symptom discomfort and pain. In such cases, the social workers' efforts would be directed toward minimizing emotional stress because the relationship between stress and the perception of pain is well known.

It is a truism that psychological and social factors are important in the care of the ill child and must always be taken into consideration. The relationship of these factors to outcome of treatment is not well documented. However, studies done in England concluded that young children whose mothers stayed with them in the hospital had fewer postoperative incidence of infection and hemorrhage than those whose mothers did not room-in (Stacey and Hall, 1979, p. 23). These findings suggest that an increased sense of security in the patient may lessen the incidence of postoperative complications. It is to be hoped that such studies will be replicated at other centers in order to confirm these results.

Response to illness and hospitalization varies, depending on the age of the child and other factors. For example, in the young child, separation anxiety is the primary fear. For the adolescent, at work on developmental tasks, such as issues of independence vs. dependence, the passive role of the patient and attendant loss of autonomy pose a threat to his shaky identity.

The often unspoken fear of the seriously ill child is the fear of dying. We know from Kübler-Ross and others, and from our own experiences, that children have different concepts of death, depending on age and individual experiences. "...Up to the age of three, a child is concerned only about separation, later followed by a fear of mutilation. It is at this age that the small child begins to mobilize, to take his first trips out into the world..(he) may see the first beloved pet run over...this is what mutilation means to him...concern about the integrity of his body...Death is not a permanent fact for the three- to five-year-old. It is temporary as burying a flower bulb into the soil in the fall, to have it come up again the following spring..." (Kübler-Ross, 1969, p. 178). A young urology patient attended a children's group meeting during a hospitalization when he was only five and asked, "If I die and go to Heaven, when I get well, can I come back?"

Children from about the age of ten have a pretty accurate concept of the finality of death. According to Morrisey "...Death-anxiety may be present in children, at least those hospitalized with catastrophic illness, much more frequently than some authors believe" (Parad, 1965, p. 331). He cites incidents of death-anxiety in children as young as three and a half. What those of us who are working with these children can do is facilitate the child's expression of his fears through projective play, group therapy, or individual therapy. It is necessary, of course, to involve the parents and to discuss with them how much they wish to tell the child about his illness and to share our own recommendations, if requested.

There does not seem to be consensus regarding how to answer the fatally ill child who asks directly or indirectly, "Am I going to die?" After one has assessed how much the child already knows, the medical realities, the family's coping capacities, and the child's own emotional needs and strength, one is still faced with the question, "Can a child deal with the fact of his own impending death — a task which tests all the adaptive and emotional strengths of most adults?" There is general agreement that the child already knows on some level even before he asks the question or at least suspects. Denial on the part of the family and professional leaves him feeling abandoned and alone with his fears. There are those who feel with Morrisey that, "While one would not inform a fatally ill child of his diagnosis or prognosis, the stricken child also has his own fearful concepts regarding the nature of death, and may have numerous clues that something strange and terrible is happening to him" (Parad, 1965, p. 325). It is toward the amelioration of those fearful concepts that therapy should be geared.

Dr. Lindy Burton has written the following:

> ...Clinicians vary as to the advice they offer. Some advocate that the child should be told, and emphasize the relief experienced by children with whom the diagnosis was discussed. They argue that mothers who decide not to tell use all their available emotional energy in the negative and largely unsuccessful pursuit of hiding the diagnosis, rather than in the more positive task of supporting the child....Many adults — parents and medical personnel alike — tend to deny that young children are aware of

the implications of their illness...it may result from an understandable unwillingness to accept the fact that the child must cope not only with the physical aspects of his illness, but also with the concomitant emotional distress....Parents may be helped to cope with the pain that such thoughts occasion by being challenged "to protect their child from the knowledge that his lifespan is limited". The child should be surrounded by a sense of security...security enables the child to "face unsafety," unsafety being either "the knowledge of their approaching death...apprehensions concerning investigations or treatment, changes in the situation, hospital admission, or the acceptance of increasing weakness."

In addition, "security does what deceptions or denial cannot do—it protects from that isolation that accentuates all suffering" (1974, p. 22).

In all cases, the role of hope cannot be overemphasized, and it is applicable both to the patient and his parents. Friedman comments: "...Unlike massive denial, hope does not interfere with effective behavior, and was entirely compatible with an intellectual acceptance of reality" (Burton, p. 22). Kübler-Ross on the same note says, "...It is this glimpse of hope which maintains them (patients) through days, weeks or months of suffering....No matter what we call it, we found that all our patients maintained a little bit of it and were nourished by it in especially difficult times. They showed the greatest confidence in the doctors who allowed for every hope—realistic or not—and appreciated it when hope was offered in spite of bad news" (1969, p. 139).

The study of Friedman et al., which focuses on parents of children with neoplastic disease, contains a pertinent observation relative to children: "Our impression is that *some* acknowledgment of the illness is often helpful, especially in the older child, in preventing the child from feeling isolated believing that others are not aware of what he is experiencing, or feeling that his disease is 'too awful' to talk about" (Parad, 1965, p. 325).

For the child, the hospital is a frightening place even if a parent rooms in, though this helps. Separated from familiar surroundings, often not understanding the reason for painful treatment procedures, subjected to dreaded finger sticks for blood, immobilized by having to stay in bed, fearing they will not be able to get the nurse's attention, and (for the chronically or seriously ill child) wondering, "Can they help me?" children confront hospitalization as a perilous journey.

There is an even higher level of anxiety around G.U. problems because the genital area is often involved. Sanger and Petrillo note that "...regardless of age a child will have castration fears from procedures involving the genitals...." (1972, p. 222). Symptoms such as incontinence and painful urination can be a source of embarrassment and discomfort, and tests can be invasive and frightening, i.e. catheterization, an IVP (intravenous pyelogram). Frequently a tube must be inserted into the bladder, and postoperatively the child might experience painful bladder spasms.

In weekly Children's Group Meetings on the Pediatric Urology Service,* many of these fears surfaced and we were able to deal with them. Children facing surgery were afraid they might wake up in the middle of the operation or that they would never wake up. A boy of latency age was concerned that he might say or do something crazy while under anesthesia. A little girl, terrified of having blood drawn, expressed the concern that all her blood might run out. Fears of mutilation were expressed in dreams, such as that of a boy of ten who told of a dream where the doctors were chasing him with a knife. Puppet play permitted a safe outlet for anger the children felt with their plight.

Many factors influence how a child adjusts to hospitalization. Some relate to the child, i.e. his age, personality, and experiences prior to hospitalization; others relate to his family as a unit, i.e. how they have coped with past life-crisis events, the mother-child relationship, and so forth. Still other factors seem to be outside the family and independent of it, such as hospital policy and organizational structure, general attitude of health-care personnel toward patients, and (in the case of the chronically ill patient) how the doctor and the child's parents negotiate his "health career." These latter concepts are explored in studies by a group of medical sociologists in England (Stacey and Hall, 1979).

For our purpose, certain of their findings seem worthy of note. For example, one of the researchers found that those children for whom hospitalization was the most stressful, whom he calls the most vulnerable, had had limited socializing, had recently had an upsetting experience, such as starting school, and had overanxious mothers. He is working on more refined tests to detect the vulnerable child so that remedial action can be started in advance of hospitalization. This would be of special value for elective admissions.

Another finding of the same medical sociologists is that there is a

---

*Babies Hospital, Columbia-Presbyterian Medical Center, New York, New York.

correlation between the child's perception of his situation (his understanding of why he is in the hospital and how much faith he has in the help of the treatment) and his adjustment to hospitalization. While this particular study was done with adolescents, my own experience with younger children confirms that if children can make some sense of why they are in the hospital, they tend to be more cooperative and less anxious. The importance of the role of hope is relevant here. The child without hope for whom the hospitalization seems purposeless is depressed and uncooperative and may respond less favorably to treatment than children with more confidence in their hospitalization.

In the same study the author (Clough) states that we tend to label children as *spoiled* or *uncooperative* when they do not adjust well to hospitalization but "...such labels fail to do justice to the patient's serious endeavors to find meaning and purpose in their situation, to establish hope and to overcome fear" (Stacey and Hall, p. 81).

On the Pediatric G.U. Service we have a multifaceted program geared to lessening the stress of our patients and their families and to providing needed support. The Children's Group Meetings, previously mentioned, serve the purpose of ventilation, sharing of information, and mutual support. A child psychiatrist and the social worker are co-therapists for this group as well as for a parallel group for parents. Children share coping techniques for dealing with needles, talk of their concerns about procedures, such as having catheters inserted, and talk about dread of operations, loneliness, and mundane issues, such as wanting double portions of favorite foods or objecting to early light-out because of the bedtime of younger children.

Since knowledge is a good antidote against fear, we have also prepared a booklet for our children entitled: "Snippy's Coloring Book About the Things They Do to You in the Hospital." It is amply illustrated and written in simple language to explain some of the common urologic procedures that Snippy (who looks a lot like Snoopy) undergoes.

Nurses do pre-op teaching so that children will know what to expect, and if a child is very fearful I will go with him to operating room. Liaison teaching to medical students by child psychiatrist and social worker about psychological and social components in pediatric urology is also a part of our program. The Exstrophy Support Team is available over the longer term for services to children and families.

For the parents, a group setting offers the opportunity to share concerns with others who are "in the same boat." Group support has great value to troubled parents as does sharing of coping strategies. Stresses to the marital relationship, brought on by the child's illness, are a common theme, and so is the opposite—"We've grown closer through all this."

In a large, sometimes impersonal, medical center, it is frequently the social worker who serves as friend, counselor, and advocate. In the case of chronic illness, she maintains contact with patient and family after discharge from the hospital, often mobilizing community services and supports. In the event of rehospitalization, she is there—a familiar face and friend. As a child said, "Everybody needs somebody to be there." This continuity has a reassuring effect.

Under stress, patients of all ages tend to revert to earlier coping patterns that have worked in the past in handling anxiety. At the same time, we know that crisis situations offer the potential for growth, for discovering new ways of coping when old patterns no longer work. The ego strengths thus accrued are then available for meeting future challenges more effectively. Our task is to help promote mastery of this most difficult crisis, a major illness, not only to lessen immediate discomfort and suffering but to encourage ego development and to avoid posthospital emotional symptoms. To quote from Burton—

> ...Some children not only emerge from their experiences emotionally unscathed (from hospitalization for serious illness) but actually appear strengthened as a result. Jessner, commenting on the integrative processes that can take place as a result of childhood illness, said "Illness may not only spur maturation but also widen the horizon, bring forth a greater depth of feeling, capacity for empathy and for sublimation".... Because of this any assessment of the way in which children face up to their illness must consider both the situations which threaten the child's psychological well-being, and the ways in which he attempts to overcome these threats (1974, p. 26).

By the conjoint efforts of health-care personnel we can hope to intervene positively to help the child to overcome these threats.

From the social worker, early intervention and social assessment of patient and family followed by application of appropriate helping modalities are required. These might involve crisis intervention, family counseling, individual therapy, group therapy, mobilization of community and family resources, help with practical problems, or just being there for support when needed. A cooperative relationship with medical staff, nursing, special therapists, and ancillary services, such as playroom staff, teachers, dieticians, is assumed.

Others in the joint effort are the urologist, who takes the time to explain to the child, in language he can understand, the purpose of the surgery and how it will help him and who then answers his questions; the nurse, assigned to patient instead of tasks, using dolls and teaching devices to help the child better understand and cope with scheduled procedures; the anesthesiologist, who explains that he will be with the child in the operating room to assure that he stays "asleep" until the operation is over and, when possible, offers the child a choice between the mask or a needle to put him to sleep; the playroom specialist, who knows the value of helping the sick child experience pleasure and a sense of accomplishment, using play materials creatively and bringing supplies to the bedridden child, appropriate for his age and physical condition.

Also taking part are the dietician, who manages to come up with a child's favorite food, on the permissible list; the teacher, who helps the hospitalized child maintain intellectual mastery, despite physical infirmities and who grants the child the option to decline these services; the paraverbal therapist (if the hospital is fortunate enough to have one of the practitioners of this innovative therapy on its staff), who, through the creative use of song, rhythms, movement, helps the ill child express what he cannot put into words; and the psychiatric nurse, the liaison child psychiatrist, and the social worker, who are concerned with the child's emotional adjustment to his illness. All are contributing individually and conjointly to helping the child in his effort to master the stresses and realities of serious illness.

Since hospitalization even with the best of care remains an emotionally hazardous experience, some alternatives are being explored. In England, pediatric home nursing is provided in some areas to care for children who otherwise would require hospitalization. Similar programs have been started in this country on a trial basis. This kind of care seems to be a preferred alternative in certain cases.

Home care has been suggested by Burton for terminally ill children: "Some pediatricians advocate either a program of parental participation in hospital nursing care, or the child's attendance on an out-patient basis. This need is especially pressing if the child is in the terminal state of his illness, giving parents and child a chance to experience each other as fully as possible before the final separation" (1974, p. 27).

Stacey, in *Beyond Separation* (a study in depth of children's reactions to hospitalization), sees the attitudes and forces contributing to children's distress as being so manifold, not the least of which is the clinical detachment that she ascribes to the traditional biomedical model of health care, that only drastic measures can bring about the needed changes. She writes, "What we are trying to do is address ourselves to an entire system of knowledge and to suggest how it might be modified in the better interest of the patients. Our findings call for radical reappraisal and not the simple addition of new techniques" (1979, p. 188).

I do not share her pessimistic view, but I am in agreement with her stated aim "...that unnecessary suffering should not be caused to children in the course of treating an ailment." I would add to this our concern to enhance the quality of life of the sick child and his family, if possible.

When I become discouraged with how much still needs to be done for our sick children, I try to remember where we have come from. This is well illustrated by two anecdotes taken from our group meetings. A father, at a parents' group meeting, told of having had a nephrectomy when he was sixteen. "Do you know how I found out I was going to have a kidney removed?" he asked. "The orderly who was rolling me to the operating room told me!"

At another group meeting, a mother and the grandfather began to talk to each other about the time when as a child she had had a tonsillectomy. "Pop, you told me that you were taking me to a party and instead you took me to the hospital. You know, I've been afraid of hospitals ever since."

We have come a long way toward making the hospital experience a more honest and supportive one for children, but we still have a long way to go.

References

Burton, L.: *Care of the Child Facing Death.* London and Boston, Routledge and Kegan Paul, 1974.

Kübler-Ross, E.: *On Death and Dying*. New York, Macmillan Company, 1969.
McCollum, A.T.: *Coping with Prolonged Health Impairment in Your Child*. Boston, Little, Brown and Company, 1975.
Parad, H.J. (Ed.): *Crisis Intervention: Selected Readings*. New York, Family Service Association of America, 1965.
Petrillo, M., and Sanger, S.: *Emotional Care of Hospitalized Children: An Environmental Approach*. Philadelphia, J.B. Lippincott, Co., 1972.
Stacey, M., and Hall, D. (Eds.): *Beyond Separation: Further Studies of Children in Hospital*. London and Boston, Routledge and Kegan Paul, 1979.

Chapter 23

THE CHILD WITH UROLOGIC CANCER

Terry W. Hensle

THE child dying of cancer engenders different things from the different people who cross his or her path. This special child is usually loved by his family, excessively wondered about by strangers, and largely ignored by his physicians. The terminally ill child very frequently does not receive the proper sympathetic understanding and expertise needed in meeting emotional demands and may encounter isolation and depersonalization. It is our sincere effort to interrupt the conspiracy of silence and interact with this special child during the period of his terminal illness.

Therapy

Although startling advances have been made in the therapy of many childhood tumors, including nephroblastoma (Wilm's tumor), rhabdomyosarcoma, and acute lymphatic leukemia, the great majority of children with malignant disease will die of their tumor. The current tendency, of course, is to equate excellence in medical care with aggressiveness of investigation and therapy. This is the natural outcome of the recent rapid expansion in the field of oncology. Frequently, the failure to recognize that further investigation and active treatment may be inappropriate in the presence of advanced disease has resulted in unnecessary suffering for the child. We too often fail to recognize that the capacity to act does not in itself justify the action.

When we design a therapeutic protocol for any of these children, we must keep in mind that unproven therapeutic modalities are only justifiable as part of a carefully designed, supervised clinical trial, and that any treatment plan must take into consideration the attendant morbidity to both the child and the family.

When palliative care becomes the only appropriate goal, further investigation should be carried out only if it leads to symptomatic improvement, and investigations for research purposes are justifiable only with the informed consent of the parent. In general, the physician's need to treat the child with terminal oncologic disease as well as the family's need to treat this child are unacceptable rationales for therapy. Often it is better to make an attempt at controlling the symptoms and assist the patient in living as comfortably and happily as possible, rather than trying to affect a disease process that cannot be controlled by our present medical facilities.

The treatment most often appropriate in dealing with the dying child and his family revolves around the treatment of chronic pain, dealing with the inherent fear of dying, and treatment of the mental distress involved in terminal illness.

The Management of Chronic Pain

In dealing with chronic pain in the terminally ill child one must first clarify the cause of the pain in order to make any logical step toward controlling it. Chronic pain differs from acute pain in that it has no defined beginning and end. It is usually characterized as a vicious cycle with no set time limit. The fear of pain leads to anxiety, depression, insomnia, all of which accentuate the physical components of pain. In addition to the total nature of chronic pain, it also painfully reminds the child with advanced malignant disease of his prognosis and further accentuates his agony.

The aim of managing chronic pain is to anticipate and to prevent the pain rather than to treat it. This, of course, requires regular administration of appropriate amounts of analgesics, specifically titrated against the patient's needs. There is no place for "PRN" medication orders in the treatment of chronic pain, since the roller coaster effect of recurring pain results in unnecessary suffering and the escalation of analgesic doses. The oral administration of analgesics also can allow the patient to retain a degree of independence and mobilty that is impossible when analgesics are given parenterally. Cachexia may also make regular intermuscular injections difficult and painful.

Fear of Dying

There are many common fears involved in terminal illness for both adults and children. Fear of pain, of course, is very realistic; however, to most of these children, the fear of parental loss is almost as strong. Frequently, the child will express anxiety over what his parents will do after he or she dies. Another important fear is that of isolation. The patient with advancing disease often encounters decreasing interest and few visits by his physician, members of the nursing staff, and friends from home. This must be counteracted with frequent reassurances by those in charge of his medical care to be sure that he feels he is still functional and that people are aware of him. In children with urologic cancers, the threat to body image and the concept of self often emerge as an overwhelming fear. Exentrative surgery and the frequent necessity for urinary stomas act to enhance this fear in most children with urologic oncologic disease.

Uncertainty leads to anxiety. The reluctance on the part of both family and physician to discuss the reality of the situation often enhances the child's fear. A candid, honest and supportive approach to the reality facing the patient will produce less anxiety and in the long run will be more helpful than well-intentioned dishonesty and lack of communication.

Mental Distress of Terminal Illness

The terminally ill child goes through many mental aberrations in order to deal with his disease process. These can include denial, anger, bargaining, depression, and finally acceptance. Whatever the sequence in any given patient, one can usually find a subtle balance between a realistic acceptance on one hand and a simultaneous rejection on the other. The terminally ill child not only has to accept adaptation to this situation, but also to a series of losses: school, friends, strength, physical and mental capacity, plans for the future, and ultimately life itself. The patient's family may go through similar adjustments, and an understanding of this process will assist the physician in accepting the anger of the patient or the family toward both the child's illness and the surrounding care structure.

These symptoms of mental distress often call for a thorough understanding of the dynamics of the situation by the primary physician, but they also call for outside psychological help from a hospital psychologist or psychiatrist particularly versed in the problems of death and dying.

Conclusions

The shifting symptom complexes and diminishing resources of the terminally ill child require regular and frequent reassurance for symptom control. Such practices by those providing medical care for the child will pay rich dividends in avoiding potentially serious problems and unnecessary hospitalization. The implied message that the physician has a continuing interest in the patient's welfare is a reassuring factor of major importance to both patient and family. It is interesting to note that a physician's visit will be remembered as being longer in duration and of greater meaning if the physician sits at the bedside so there is eye contact on the same level. Touching the patient, in general, brings with it reassurance. The key, then, is to develop the sensitivity to meet the patients at their level both physically and emotionally, rather than attempting to bring the patient unrealistically to a level that he or she will never again achieve.

Chapter 24

CHILDREN WITH UROLOGIC PROBLEMS: PSYCHOLOGICAL NEEDS

KATHERINE F. JETER

CHILDREN born with urologic problems are special. They have malleable egos, fragile personalities, and very anxious parents, and they deserve systematic and conscientious care. We must indeed understand them. Sigmund Freud said, "I would advise you to set aside your therapeutic ambitions and try to understand what is happening, and when you've done that, therapeutics will take care of itself." I would like to take a theoretical but practical look at this group of children and the way they are going to grow. They are going to develop first as normal children, but they have additional problems that require attention. There is every reason that children with urological diseases should be severely traumatized by what has happened to them. But we do not have any hard data, just our observations.

What are we talking about? Exstrophy of the bladder is one example. The bladder is on the outside of the body, turned wrong side out. The ureteral orifices are exposed and drip urine continuously. The genitalia will always be malformed, even after repair. In the case of a boy, the penis is splayed wide open, and no matter how elegant the reconstruction, there will always be a peculiar looking penis that he is going to live with.

Then there is "Prune-Belly" syndrome, the absence of abdominal musculature. This absence of abdominal muscles causes the abdomen to look like a prune. In the case of a baby with a patent urachus, the urine is coming out of the umbilicus. During childhood, the children with prune belly cannot be bound to hold in all those abdominal contents because this will compromise their respiratory function. So the parents have to deal with the appearance of it and to adjust to it, just as the children do. It's an obvious and apparent defect to friends and family.

Then, there is an innocuous-looking scar, which is the closure of spina bifida or meningomyelocele. The closing of a spinal defect is the opening of a Pandora's box, with problems that plague the practitioner, family, educational facilities, and friends.

Eric Erikson helped everyone see that the life-style and life process are dynamic from birth until death. He said that in the period prior to adulthood, the first ego task is the development of a sense of trust. If an infant is not able to develop a sense of trust, then he will forever be shackled by a sense of mistrust. According to Erikson's framework, you *can* go back a little, make up for what you lost, and start over again. For our purposes, the task in the first eighteen months of a child's life is the development of a sense of trust. If, because of this child's medical condition, trust does not develop, it is our responsibility to encourage an environment to make up for this.

Between the ages of two and three is the time also for the development of autonomy. Without this, there is shame and doubt. The terrible twos are a time of fantasy and a period when children realize they are boy or girl because we tell them "pretty girl" or "handsome boy." We might have to take them to the operating room for cystoscopies or a catheterization. Many children fear that some awful demon is going to go in that pipe, or that they are going to emerge from the procedure as a different sex. The problem gets bigger as the child grows older.

For preschoolers, according to Erikson, the task is to develop a sense of initiative. Without it, there is a sense of guilt. School must promote a sense of industry. The alternative is inferiority. In adolescence comes that awful struggle for identity: Who am I and where am I going? Without it, role confusion results.

Those who know parents who have given birth to a defective child see horrible disappointment because nine months of expectation and hopes have been shattered in one brief moment. That discrepancy must be resolved. There are mothers who really don't like their babies. Are we brave enough to allow them to talk about it? There are some babies who, according to research, do not particularly like their mothers.

A fantasy is shared by many parents, even those with advanced degrees. They think that if a little boy can't urinate through his penis, that penis is going to do what Aunt Maude's arm did after it became paralyzed, it will shrivel up from disuse. The fantasy may be so much a part of parents' ideas that they won't ask about it. We did an informal observation on babies at bathtime. Many of the children were incontinent for one reason or another. After the age of two or three, we found that during bathtime those children never touched their genitals. How sad it is. I have no explanation. Does the child think the genitals are broken? Does he think the parts don't work? Has something happened to cause lack of sensation?

During the course of one year, three little girls, who were born as males with cloacal exstrophy, were referred to me. It was decided that there was no possibility of constructing any male genitalia. Gender reassignment was the preferred method of treatment. Everyone was in agreement, even the parents. But one mother wrote, "You know, Micki always wants to go hunting with her daddy. Her daddy wants to take her to play racketball and she's only six. Mrs. Jeter, she's never played with a doll; I know her real sex is showing through." There's nothing in the world that I can say to Micki's mom. I can listen, empathize, and counsel, and help everyone on her care team be cognizant of what this mother is going through.

What are we going to do about three-, four-, and five-year-olds for whom we have cared and for whom mother and daddy have this incredible investment? To let go is frightening. One of the mothers said, "You know, so much time and energy have been invested in my child. Doctor Brown has operated three times, and if I let Tommy go out and hurt himself, what would he say!" Parents have to make a philosophical reckoning. Are they going to have their kids stand and watch the stream of life go by? Are they going to pitch in and put the kids in the mainstream? It's a tough decision. But it's a decision that must be made, because the child without initiative is not prepared to go much further in his social development. These young children groove on heroes. Ladies and men in white are just as good as Superman® and Plasticman. Children can be enlisted to help carry trays, push strollers, become involved. You can interact with them. It's very important when they express love to you because for the very first time they're expressing love beyond their family. (This should not be passed off as a childish expression.)

When the kids go off to school, they face a culture all its own. School is for the development of a sense of industry. "Now that I know that I can, I'm going to show you what I can do." Many children are put into special schools, not because they need it but because no one knows what to do with them in the regular schools. It's an arbitrary decision. More than anything, these children need as normal a life as possible. If they do have other problems and they do go to a regular school, it is imperative to create compensatory activities that give them the strength, courage, and tools they need.

In adolescence, incontinence and the associated problems are very serious. What kind of identity can a child develop with this kind of handicap? It's important to be like everyone else. Perhaps the adolescent tries to avoid responsibilities at school and at home. It's difficult not to permit this kind of behavior. Parents need help and support.

Children who have urologic problems may be terrified that they'll be unable to perform sexually or that something awful will happen. Girls often don't know that the vagina is different from the urethra. They have heard about that stricture and that closing up. ("If that thing is closed up, is that other thing closed up?") A physician once shocked a group of professionals when he mentioned a suggestion he gave to teenage boys. He encouraged the boys to go downtown, hire themselves a lady, and say, "I'm going to lay it on the line. I've got a problem and I'm willing to pay $40 because I want to know if I can perform." I'm not so sure that this is not a marvelous idea. If we can have surrogate sex partners for normally dysfunctional people, what's wrong with surrogate sex partners for kids who question their ability to perform? The girls all want to know if they can have babies. They don't know half the time whether they've got a uterus or not, or they don't know what it is. Some of them aren't menstruating, and some are menstruating abnormally.

The questions are always real and urgent. Who is going to answer them? In many states and cities, sex education consists of "the film" and "the book." Mothers and dads say that they tell all about sex. Most kids don't want to know about sex from their parents because they don't want to know that parents do these things; however, they sure would like to know about it from someone else.

They'd like to know how you do it and how long it takes. There's not a thing wrong with the orderly who sits down and talks to the boy with a question. What isn't all right is that there are not enough orderlies, physicians, nurses, social workers, counselors, and volunteers who are comfortable enough with sex to elicit questions and to spend the time to answer them.

Author's note: This chapter was transcribed from a taped lecture.

Chapter 25

PSYCHOSOCIAL PROBLEMS OF THE CHILD AND FAMILY UNDERGOING DIALYSIS AND TRANSPLANTATION

Morris J. Schoeneman

END-STAGE renal disease, like other chronic illnesses of childhood, constitutes a major stress for the child and family (Grushkin et al., 1973). Two important concepts should be considered in preparing a child for this stress and in developing management and rehabilitation programs (Stubblefield, 1974, p. 509). First, chronic illness inevitably produces depression, with the usual phases of emotional shock, apathy, and detachment, and the various regressive processes associated with mourning. Naturally, these responses are muted, disguised, and often appear in very subtle nonverbal and verbal communications. Second, chronic illness has a negative effect on the child's self-esteem and personal self-image. It seems evident that the healthy child is presented with a series of frustrations and disappointments as he goes through the various developmental periods and that he masters many of these experiences by relying on the hope and expectation that he will be older, stronger, and better able to solve the particular problems. The child with chronic illness, however, is likely to have more doubts about his skills, abilities, and potential for solving future problems.

This chapter will present the physical and psychosocial problems of chronic renal insufficiency (CRI) encountered by children and their families, including the stresses unique to chronic dialysis and transplantation. It will describe methods which are being used in an attempt to provide preparation and support for children and families who are about to face or have already encountered these problems. Finally, it will summarize results gained by several centers that use these methods in the physical and psychosocial rehabilitation of children with chronic renal failure.

An understanding of the problems facing children with CRI requires a discussion of the physical consequences of renal failure. Normal renal functioning encompasses four major areas: maintenance of homeostasis of the body fluids, electrolytes and acid-base balance; excretion of the accumulated waste products of nitrogen metabolism; endocrine functioning through production of active metabolites of Vitamin D for normal bone structure and Erythropoietin for normal red blood cell production; and maintenance of normal growth, sexual maturation, and neuromuscular function. Renal insufficiency ultimately leads to defects in all of these areas.

Conservative management of CRI involves dietary and pharmacologic manipulations to prevent or ameliorate these problems. When renal insufficiency is so advanced that these measures are inadequate, chronic dialysis (either hemo or peritoneal dialysis) or renal transplantation are required. Dialysis and transplantation are now well beyond the experimental stage and are commonly applied to children suffering from CRI who would otherwise be doomed to death. Approximately four children per million population require the initiation of chronic dialysis or transplantation yearly (Mauer, 1978, p. 489). These procedures, although lifesaving, impose heavy physical and psychosocial costs on the patients and their families. Even though the technical problems involved in the care of children and adolescents with CRI are in general similar to those in adults, the physical and psychological development intrinsic to the growing child poses management difficulties that are quite different from those of adult patients (Korsch et al., 1973).

The physical costs include cosmetic defects caused by the illness itself, by side effects of medications, and by surgical procedures. For example, CRI usually produces some degree of muscle wasting and often leads to short stature, bony deformities, and lack of maturation of the secondary sexual characteristics. Side effects of the immunosuppressive medications used to treat the underlying disease or to maintain a renal transplant include production of Cushingoid facies, acne, hirsutism, alopecia, striae, and cataracts. Surgical procedures cause pain and produce undesirable scars, external shunts, and stomas. Urinary leakage is often a source of odor and embarrassment. Finally, these children are keenly aware of a decrease in their physical strength and endurance, and are constantly irritated by their restricted diets and activity levels.

Psychosocial costs are imposed in several ways. Patients are constantly anxious about the possibility of impending pain, invasive procedures, loss of dialysis access, serious illness, and death. They live under the continuing threat of surgical removal of parts of their bodies: both kidneys, spleen, and parathyroid glands. They also have the constant worry concerning early posttransplant complications and early and late transplant loss due to immunological rejection. They must contend with disruption of their school life and social life because of the demands of travel time back and forth to the hospital for evaluations, dialysis, and occasional long-term hospitalizations. In addition, dietary restrictions, limitation of activity, cosmetic defects, and lack of physical growth and sexual development greatly limit their social maturation and peer relationships. Finally, family disruption is induced by pressures of finances and by time and energy expenditures.

As a result of these physical and psychosocial problems, certain types of psychological coping mechanisms and psychopathology commonly appear (Grushkin et al., 1973; Korsch and Raimbault, 1973; Fine et al., 1970; Korsch et al., 1971; Primack et al., 1976; Primack and Greifer, 1977; Bouras et al., 1976). With careful observation, the initial phases of these reactions can be identified as soon as the child and family are made aware of the diagnosis of chronic renal disease, long before the need for dialysis and transplant occurs. Among the patients, there is an initial period of evident anxiety and depression. Gradually, mobilization of defenses introduces strong denial, reaction formation, projection, displacement, and isolation of affect. In spite of, or perhaps as a consequence of, these protective mechanisms, most children develop a constriction of personality and a withdrawal from interest in outside events and peer relationships. Intellectual functioning drops below actual potential and school truancy becomes a common occurrence. These problems are compounded by the development of a poor self-image that, especially in adolescents, leads to a lack of interest in planning for a future social and sexual role. Guilt is an overriding concern of these patients; many feel that bad behavior on their part has led to their illness, and some suspect that treatment failures, and especially transplant losses, are somehow their fault. Dependence on machines, hospital staff, and family for life support inhibits the normal development of independence and separation from family that is a part of normal maturation. Parents and staff often become overprotective, and the children generally acquiesce with this situation. Some patients, especially adolescents, manage to rebel against such smothering, but unfortunately they often manifest their rebellion as noncompliance with diet, medications, school attendance, or appearance for dialysis treatments. The occasional ultimate expression of defiance and noncompliance is suicide.

The effect of chronic renal failure on the family is often disrupting. Long-lasting anxiety, fear, depression, sibling rivalry, and overprotectiveness are almost universal. Depending on the pre-illness family structure, the problem of the uremic child can lead to increasing discord and parental separation, or can produce strong unification of parents and siblings around the chronically ill child. In cases of transplant donation by a parent or sibling, graft failure produces intense guilt and sorrow in the donor and the recipient. Family members undergo intense stress deciding whether to attempt kidney donation to their child or sibling.

How can one best prepare a child and its family for the stresses of CRI, dialysis, and transplant in order to avoid or at least ameliorate these problems? Attempts have been made by several groups that care for children with chronic renal disease to apply preventive and supportive measures early in the course (Grushkin et al., 1973; Korsch et al., 1973; Korsch and Raimbault, 1973; Fine et al., 1978; Korsch et al., 1978). A most important point is to begin working with the patient and family from the time of diagnosis of a disease that is known to progress to chronic renal failure. The natural history of the disease, as modified by treatment, must be described, with frequent review and with time allowed for repeated questioning. The physical and psychosocial costs to be expected are brought to the family's attention early in the course. Support and education must be given on a continuing basis to the child and family, and specific problems, e.g. dietary management, transportation, schooling, insurance, and so forth, must be anticipated and managed by knowledgeable professionals. So far, the best results are reported by groups that have set up a psychosocial support team (Korsch and Raimbault, 1973; Korsch et al., 1978). Such a team generally consists of a pediatric nephrologist, vascular and urologic surgeons, in-patient nursing and dialysis nursing representatives, public health or visiting nurse representatives, a hospital teacher, a social worker, a psychologist and/or psychiatrist, a dietician, a play therapist, and a physical therapist. A successful team effort is based on giving continuous support and education to each patient and family and also to the group of involved physicians, nurses, and paramedical personnel. Team members meet with each other in sensitivity sessions at regular intervals to discuss openly their feelings about each other, their own various means of handling problems, and the best course of action for individual children. Input from the children, parents, and other siblings is obtained at other meetings. Team members are often responsible for arranging and being present at adolescent group meetings, meetings of several families of children on dialysis or transplant, and introductory meetings of a new patient with a child and family already on chronic dialysis or transplant. Typical problems handled by individual members of the team include preparing a preschooler for the trauma of vascular access surgery or nephrectomy, helping an adolescent with applications to college or job interviews, and helping a family finance the automobile needed to bring the child to the hospital for dialysis several times a week. The success of such a team effort is just beginning to be evaluated.

Another approach has been reported by Greifer et al. (Primack et al., 1976; Primack and Greifer, 1977). They sent children on chronic dialysis and transplantation to sleep-away camp equipped with a dialysis unit. A recreational program was developed that integrated the uremic children with their normal peers. The expectation was that self-esteem and physical endurance might improve and that families would appreciate some time away from the child's immediate medical problems.

Studies of the results of comprehensive psychosocial team intervention with children with chronic renal failure and their families are few. The only formal studies available are of children and families who have been through the process of CRI and have had a successful renal transplant (Korsch et al., 1973; Korsch and Raimbault, 1973; Fine et al., 1978; Korsch et al., 1978). The data in these studies were collected using several personality tests, such as The California Test of Personality and the Piers-Harris Self-Esteem Scale, as well as several tests that explore body image in a less structured and verbal manner, such as the Draw-a-Person Test and the Draw-What's-Inside-the-Person Test. Control children for these evaluations were taken from a normal population and a group of children with other kinds of chronic diseases. The results in forty-one children, five years after successful renal transplantation, show that total personality score was not significantly different from that of normals. Most children and families returned to their preillness levels of adaptation and the children had the usual types of social and emotional problems expected for their age group. Eighty-seven percent of these patients were involved in some kind of meaningful activity, including return to full-time schooling (college, graduate school, and professional school), jobs, and marriage (with successful childbearing). However, an analysis of subscores of the testing showed that social adjustment was significantly decreased compared to normal controls, specifically with restriction in socialization and social activity. Also, self-esteem was significantly lower than in normal controls. More worrisome is the finding that noncompliance with medications, especially steroids, was present in eight of the forty-one children (Korsch et al., 1978). Most were adolescent girls who showed extreme denial, rebellion, and depression, and were specifically upset about the cosmetic side effects of their medication. Noncompliance led to loss of the transplant and a return to chronic dialysis in each of these patients. Features found to be common to the noncompliant population, and whose recognition may be useful for prevention, included extremely deviant scores on personality tests, low family income, absent father, and poor communication among family members measured by family function testing. Attempts are underway to find ways of improving patient and family support so that social adjustment, self-esteem, and compliance may be enhanced.

The summer camp experience described by Greifer et al. provides a more optimistic viewpoint. Twenty-four children on chronic hemodialysis were compared to seventy-six normal children. The uremic children had significantly lower scores for self-esteem (Piers-Harris Scale) than the normals at the beginning of the two-week overnight camp session. The children with CRI had a substantial improvement in self-esteem, greater than that seen in the controls, by the end of the session. In addition, later follow-up of the children's behavior with families, schools, and the home dialysis unit revealed evidence of increased independent activity, better peer relationships, increased self-care on dialysis, decreased passivity, and increased physical endurance. Families reported an increased recognition of their previous overprotective behavior and admitted to appreciating the two-week respite while the child was away at camp, allowing more time for interaction with healthy siblings.

In summary, the physical and psychosocial stresses of chronic illness in children, and specifically the stresses of CRI, dialysis, and transplantation, are a major challenge in devising methods of prevention and support. The experience with handling these problems is slowly increasing. Further innovative approaches are required and careful studies of their effectiveness are needed so that a uniform recommendation can be made for use by all centers that have undertaken the management of children with chronic renal disease.

References

Bouras, M., Silvestre, D., Broyer, M., and Raimbault, G.: Renal transplantation in children: A psychological survey. *Clinical Nephrology,* 6:478-482, 1976.

Fine, R.M., Korsch, B.M., Grushkin, C.M., and Lieberman, E.: Hemodialysis in children. *American Journal of Diseases of Children,* 119:498-504, 1970.

Fine, R.M., Malekzadeh, M.H., Pennisi, A.J., Ettinger, R.B., Uittenbogaart, C.H., Negrete, V.F., and Korsch,, B.M.: Long-term results of renal transplantation in children. *Pediatrics,* 61:641-650, 1978.

Grushkin, C.M., Korsch, B.M., and Fine, R.N.: The outlook for adolescents with chronic renal failure. *Pediatric Clinics of North America,* 20:953-963, 1973.

Korsch, B., and Raimbault, G.: Psycho-social aspects. In T. Lindholm (Ed.): *The Gambro Symposium on Paediatric Haemodialysis.* Lund, A.B. Skanska Publisher, 1973, pp. 6-169.

Korsch, B.M., Fine, R.N., Grushkin, C.M., and Negrete, V.F.: Experiences with children and their families during extended hemodialysis and kidney transplantation. *Pediatric Clinics of North America,* 18:625-637, 1971.

Korsch, B.M.., Negrete, V.F., Gardner, J.E., Weinstock, C.L., Mercer, A.S., Grushkin, C.M., and Fine, R.N.: Kidney transplantation in children: Psychosocial follow-up study on child and family. *Journal of Pediatrics,* 83:399-408, 1973.

Korsch, B.M., Fine, R.N., and Negrete, V.F.: Noncompliance in children with renal transplants. *Pediatrics,* 61:872-876, 1978.

Mauer, S.M.: Pediatric renal dialysis. In C.M. Edelmann, Jr., (Ed.): *Pediatric Kidney Disease* (Volume 1). Boston, Little, Brown and Co., 1978, p. 509.

Primack, W.A., and Greifer, I.: Summer camp hemodialysis for children with chronic renal failure. *Pediatrics,* 60:46-50, 1977.

Primack, W., Brown, P., Schoeneman, M., Goldsmith, D., and Greifer, I.: Improvement in self-concept of children on chronic hemodialysis attending a summer camp. *Proceedings of the Clinical Dialysis and Transplant Forum,* 6:35,

1976.

Stubblefield, R.L.: Psychiatric complications of chronic illness in children. In J.A. Downey and N.L. Low (Eds.): *The Child with Disabling Illness*. Philadelphia, W.B. Saunders, Co., 1974, p. 509.

IV.
PSYCHOSOCIAL CONSIDERATIONS FOR THE PATIENT AND THE FAMILY

Chapter 26

THE PATIENT'S FREEDOM IN DECISION MAKING

Bruce L. Danto

PERHAPS at no other time in history has man been surrounded by more slogans and placards and more declamations of the rights of mankind. Court dockets are filled with litigation involving contests between parties as to their rights. Bookstalls carry novels and texts with the word *right* in the title and imprinted in different colors and letter sizes on the covers. Billboards and advertisements in newspapers and magazines carry the message and implore the reader to support worthy causes ranging from "Save the Baby Seals, they have a right to live!" to "Remember, you too have a right to breathe" or "You have a right to be loved, smell good, be the best dancer on the floor," and so forth. Lost among the growing numbers of human rights and searches for freedom is that right and freedom of the cancer patient to make decisions about many areas of his treatment, care, and future.

Despite obvious disappointment, it is interesting to observe that many of the most quoted books available on the topic of death, bereavement, and the cancer patient do not deal directly with this topic. Some authors, like Glaser and Strauss (1965), discuss decision making from the perspective of members of the medical team as well as from that of the family of the cancer patient. Despite four specific references within their book to the area of decision making in general, not one dealt with the patient and how to bring him into the scene or whether he belongs in the decision scene at all.

Ignace Lepp (1968) reasons that there is a distinction between suicide and voluntary death. In this way, he approaches but does not reach the issue of a patient's freedom to make decisions. Lepp expresses an opinion that suicide differs from voluntary death. How does he explain this? He chose a model of a resistance fighter or soldier during wartime and rationalized that such a person chooses death as an outgrowth of a generous or self-sacrificing relationship with the universe. As to the suicidal person, he felt he displayed an egocentric and negative attitude in his decision to die. Although close to the issue, Lepp missed the mark as he omitted the cancer patient and became lost in a confusion of moral judgment and an insufficient understanding of the psychodynamics of suicide.

Glaser and Strauss (1965) come close to an approach to the topic of rights when they discuss the professional rights of nurses and the open and closed forms of awareness of dying on the part of the patient. It would appear to be almost too obvious to anyone that before a patient's rights can be discussed or determined it must be clear that he knows what condition he has so that he can know what he must make a decision about. As medical and hospital customs would have it, there are too many physicians who take the "easy way out" by choosing not to tell a patient that he has a cancer. Further, the nurses follow suit by rationalizing that "We are only here to serve the orders of the doctor." Thus, each member of the medical team interacts to produce closed awareness. Communication of the cancer state or the significance of special treatment ordered by the physician is subtly conveyed by hints, contradictions in orders and explanations, and motoric gestures like silent tears, averted eye contact, and hushed discussion or frequent subject changes during conversation.

Thus, as long as a conspiracy of silence and deception persists, the patient is never free to exercise any right to make a decision. As his illness reaches a state of progressive weakness and discomfort, the patient finds that he is looking for the proverbial pea under the same old three shells. Perhaps he becomes resigned to the fact that no one wants to talk to him about his concerns, suspicions, fears, hopes, and the decisions he would like to make if only he knew what the facts call for.

Usually, most patients, even the helpless and overly dependent ones, can arrive at a decision of what to do if they are given clear-cut alternatives and an analysis of what variables are constant and which ones have some flexibility. Most of the time, professional medical personnel feel that it is best to let the patient slip away from his illness and his life. They can perform their duties well and efficiently because they develop and seek refuge in the ego defenses of isolation and rationalization. Tragically, they miss an opportunity to learn from their patient, to share an important and personal experience with another human being and to feel they have humanely assisted as a life ends. They have donned the armor of programmed management and can anticipate the development of an image that is virtually indistinguishable from any other piece of hospital machinery or physical equipment. Such an image does exist in many hospital and medical settings and the need to humanize the patient-treatment relationship is just as challenging today as it was when patients were sent to the Temple of Aescalapius for divine healing, the application of soothing, aromatic oils, and the adornment of togas, which became the precursors of modern hospital patient gowns.

Ever present is the challenge of converting a mechanistic individual into a living, humanistic person, one who displays sensitivity to the feelings of others. If our approach were to achieve this goal, we would run into the fact that too many medical personnel lack this orientation. They will hear others lecture and demonstrate the art of recognizing human concerns, anxiety, and the wish to maintain self-identity by sharing in the decision-making process. Notwithstanding exposure to the "this-is-how-you-can-do-it" approach, some professionals respond in the same old, insensitive way when put to the test at the bedside. Therefore, we must ask how we can get around the problem of the insensitive professional and how we can develop an approach that assists him and the patient in regard to the patient's sharing in the decision-making process.

These goals can be achieved at the very beginning of a doctor-patient relationship. When a lesion is observed and surgical intervention and biopsy are required, the patient can be informed with or without his family being present, and he can be asked whether or not he wishes to be told all the facts. Such an approach offers him a chance to begin with making a decision.

With some lesions, there can be no options. There are tumors where the decision is primarily medical or surgical like a brain tumor, cancer of the prostate, a testicular or ovarian cancer, and others. However, the patient can be encouraged to participate in the decision-making aspects of even a purely medical decision-making issue. The patient can decide when he can be admitted for the surgical biopsy and intervention, how much he wants to be told about the exact nature of the cancer if the lesion turns out to be malignant, how he would like the news to be handled with his family, and what his role will be in the convalescent period. Most patients do not realize that they can share in decisions regarding the type of medication they receive by keeping a record of the effective dose so that their therapists will know what is happening pharmacologically. Such a prescribed activity assists the patient in another way as it gives him something to do. He assumes an active role in his treatment instead of being only the body presented for therapy and healing. Thus, the patient can become a member of the medical team and can share in the decisions that will affect his life and future.

Other decision-making opportunities are available. At some hospitals, the patient can select from the hospital's collection of such items as plants, art objects, pictures, and paintings to decorate his room. These measures can be taken to sustain the terminal patient psychologically.

Thus far, then, from the very beginning, the patient has been encouraged to participate and join members of the medical team in making different types of decisions. However, there are more areas in which his role as a decider can be seen. Once he knows that his surgeon is going to stick by him and assure him that pain and discomfort will be kept at a minimum, he can choose from among many analgesic measures that are available. As the disease progresses, such measures may include drugs, nerve blocks on a local basis, radiation therapy, hypnosis, and cordotomy. As he works through his feelings about his prognosis, he may be offered an opportunity to choose how long he wants his medical team to fight for his life, how many transfusions he should receive, for how long heroic measures should be continued, when he should be readmitted to the hospital for the final treatment phase in terms of medical supportive care, and so forth. These are areas about which he may have strong feelings, and he should be given an opportunity to express them and to participate in the decision-making process.

Some of his decisions or at least wishes may very well depend upon the feelings expressed by family members. For example, they may have a different concept of the length of time they can tolerate having the patient at home before the final terminal phase. They may have feelings also about how long life should be maintained with heroic measures during coma. Further, they may have firm ideas about how they want to see pain and discomfort relieved. What does the medical team do? Will it feel that too many cooks will spoil the broth? Wouldn't it be better if only doctors and nurses make decisions, thereby avoiding all that hassle and mixed feelings?

What the medical team must do is appreciate the fact that administrative ease is not always the best measure of appropriate functioning for anyone. As the patient and his family participate to any extent possible, the disastrous effects of anticipatory grief and bereavement can be lessened. Guilt feelings about having let the patient down are ameliorated, and broken emotional ties are made less painful. The patient becomes more accepting of the future and recognizes that to some extent he is the master of what will come. To feel that you can steer the boat is better and more supportive than to feel helpless, trapped in a routine of staring at the walls and wondering what will come next and what will be done.

The medical team can offer encouragement to the patient in other areas of his life. He can be offered assistance in the practical matters that may have been neglected—an evaluation of his estate, a review of his will or the making of a will. He should be urged to think about these areas and discuss them with his family so that provisions for those he cares about can be made. Shared decisions about the financing of children's education as well as a spouse's survivorship can be made, and professional resources for legal guidance can be obtained through members of the treatment or medical team. Questions such as whether or not a home should be sold or whether or not the surviving spouse can be encouraged to remarry are important areas that should be discussed by the patient with some member of the medical team. In these ways, the real feelings of the patient can be made known, and he can discover other ways to control and share in the decisions that will affect his life and the lives of his loved ones.

Once members of the medical team learn to recognize the extent to which the patient can make or participate in decisions about his life as a patient, they can experience a view of a patient in terms of his total life situational setting. They will be able to see beyond the limitations of a disease model/sick body concept. A growing sense of strength and closer emotional bonding will be imparted to the patient and his close family members. The reality of such an achievement is poignant and impressive.

As a cancer process approaches terminality, one of the most difficult decisions a family must make concerns the choice of a cemetery site. Recently, this author was asked to assist in just such a matter.

On the basis of previous difficulties after the fact of death, the author raised questions about the thoughts of family members concerning location in the cemetery. Certain relatives wanted the patient to be interred in their particular family plot, utilizing one of six graves. No sooner had this offer been made, than the donor felt regret, for the near-deceased voiced his desire that a large headstone be erected. The donor learned that not only would the back three gravesites of the six-grave plot be completely covered, but also that there would not be enough room for other members of his close family. Further, he was a man who felt that he had never accomplished anything in his lifetime. His one unexpressed hope for immortality rested in the thought of a headstone inscribed with his own name. After he had probably surrendered the back three graves for the dying man's headstone, he learned that the cemetery would not permit two names to appear on the same stone. He was crushed and felt that he was destined for eternal obscurity. Careful exploration brought out the facts, and the author approached the patient. The patient was too concerned about being near death to worry about "where my remains are going to be dumped. Tell cousin Herman I'd rather be near Aunt Tillie anyway. I always hated her and this way I can really annoy her." At a time of intense pain and gloom, he suddenly began to laugh about the whole thing. He found it possible to show compassion for Herman and was relieved to find some humor in his last few days of life. Unvoiced but noted by the author was the fact that among the final events of this man's life was his decision about where he wanted to be buried. This decision was based on an effort to relieve his cousin, but it was his decision and it meant that he still possessed some power and some worth; he could still make someone else's life easier.

In this chapter, the author has attempted to illustrate in practical ways how members of the medical team can encourage and direct the cancer patient to share in decision making. Such efforts include how much he wants to be told about the surgical and diagnostic findings, subjective reporting of the clinical effectiveness of analgesic and other creature-comfort medication, decisions about readmissions to the hospital, and how long his life should be supported by heroic measures. The medical team can also offer him the emotional support necessary to share decisions with his family regarding family problems, relationships, and legal matters. Finally he can express his thoughts about a place of burial, the remarriage of his spouse, the education plans of children, and other decisions to be made after his death. Throughout all of this decision-making experience, the role of the patient and medical team remains humanized, and greater dignity is achieved by their working together. The shared making of decisions will sustain the patient's sense of social attachment and will enhance the professional caregiver's degree of involvement with the patient as a person.

References

Feifel, H. (Ed.): *The Meaning of Death*. New York, McGraw-Hill Co., 1959.
Glaser, B.G., and Strauss, A.L.: *Awareness of Dying*. Chicago, Aldine Publishing Co., 1965.
Hinton, J.: *Dying*. Baltimore, Penguin Books, Inc., 1967.
Kübler-Ross, E.: *On Death and Dying*. New York, Macmillan Co., 1969.
Lepp, I.: *Death and Its Mysteries*. New York, Macmillan Co., 1968.
Schoenberg, B., et al. (Eds.): *Loss and Grief: Psychological Management in Medical Practice*. New York, Columbia University Press, 1970.

Chapter 27

ESTATE PLANNING FOR THE TERMINALLY ILL

Gerald Rosner

THERE are distinct advantages to planning an estate while the testator is in good health. Time is normally the ally of the estate planner—time to discuss, to think, to ponder, to deliberate, to make gifts, to shift income, to buy and sell assets.

Time—lack of it, that is—is the enemy when doing premortem estate planning for a terminally ill person. The job is easier if the patient is lucid. If the illness causes unremitting pain, however, and decathexis has already set in, the estate planner's task is made immeasurably more difficult, if not impossible. We will therefore assume throughout that the testator, though diagnosed as terminally ill, is in possession of his/her faculties and fully cognizant of the objectives to be accomplished.

It is generally recognized that any activity which helps one openly and truthfully come to grips with the reality of death is beneficial to a dying patient. Denial, anger, and depression often precede acceptance of mortality as the final stage of life (Kübler-Ross, 1974). While working with a dying patient, however, the estate planner is bound to identify with his client facing, perhaps for the first time, the inevitability of his own death. The trauma that can occur in such a situational crisis is dealt with at length in an article by Ann Kliman and Edward Schlesinger, titled "Counseling Your Dying Client and His Family" (1979). If the estate planner cannot cope with the concept of imminent death, he should withdraw early and assist the family in finding an estate planner who can deal with the situation on a more competent level. In this author's opinion, at least, a Chartered Life Underwriter (C.L.U.), who has been in business long enough to have handled many death claims, is often an ideal choice as estate planner to the terminally ill. Stephan Leimberg has made an important contribution to this subject in his article "Death Sensitization for the Estate Planner" (1976).

Listing the Assets

The first and most obvious task is to list the assets and liabilities. As any estate planner knows, this can be a difficult task under the best of circumstances. When dealing with a terminally ill patient, it is frequently necessary to enlist the aid of a trusted family member in finding the assets, verifying their existence and ownership from original documents, and placing a current market value on them.

The order of listing is important. I have found that starting with tangible real property when presenting the list to the testator is comforting to him or her. These are the items with which he is most familiar and to which he feels some nostalgic attachment. Contrary to conventional balance-sheet procedures, I would list cash and securities last. After real estate, I would show objects of art, coin and stamp collections, books and records.

Reviewing the asset listing with a terminally ill testator can be an emotionally charged experience. The estate planner would be well advised to ask the attending physician whether his patient is up to the ordeal and what time of day or evening would be least enervating.

It is also advisable to have the family attorney present as well as the spouse, provided the spouse is calm and level-headed. If not, another less volatile family member should be selected.

Distributing the Assets

Once the assets have been clearly identified and evaluated, every opportunity should be afforded the testator to articulate his or her own dispositive wishes. The estate planner must be a good listener. He must also be alert to body language, to gestures, to glances. He can learn as much by indirection as he can from outright response.

The terminally ill client may, as a result of his illness and/or treatment, show signs of fatigue and forgetfulness. These are not necessarily signals to stop the interview. A brief halt, a pause, may be in order. When the discussion resumes, it is advisable to recapitulate and confirm the decisions previously made.

Intrafamilial relationships must be quickly grasped by the estate planner. Conflicts, rivalries, and slights real and imagined exist in all families and are often magnified when a family member is terminally ill. They must be put in perspective.

Special circumstances, such as estrangements, retarded and otherwise disabled children and grandchildren, and irresponsible in-laws, must be recognized and confirmed by the estate planner who, as an impartial outsider, will often be favored with confidences more readily than close friends and family members.

Redoing the Last Testament

The laws of intestacy are rigid and unforgiving. It is as if they were written with a punitive intent. Hence, a carefully drawn will is critical to the estate-planning process.

After the assets have been identified and the testator's wishes made known, it is the estate planner's job to convey them to the attorney, with whom he will work closely in considering the variety of methods of distribution, weighing their impact in terms of taxes and selecting the most advantageous. Specific bequests to family members should reflect clearly the testator's expressed wishes; leaving the amounts and timing up to the executor and/or testamentary trustee is not a recommended substitute.

The testamentary act, the leaving behind of something of oneself, is the one mechanism available to all as a step in the direction of immortality. Our sons carry our names on, whether with pride or with pain cannot be foretold. Our daughters and their progeny may or may not be proud living reminders of our existence. For many, even those with large families, when faced with the reality of imminent death, some additional insurance is required. Money or other property will salve a guilt-ridden conscience, reduce anxieties, and enable us to take that last breath with less pain. If the estate planner accomplishes this much for the terminally ill patient, and nothing more, his service is a valid adjunct to the doctor's, nurse's, and minister's roles.

Choosing the Executor

The proper choice of executor is crucial to the implementation of the wishes and desires of the estate owner as they were developed by the planner and reduced to writing by the attorney.

The task of administering an estate is no easy one. In addition to coping with ever-changing business cycles, trying to predict interest rate movements and anticipating inflation or recession, an executor is obliged to conserve the estate while producing adequate income for the income beneficiaries. Such an awesome responsibility can be met only by someone with experience and skills equal to the task. That someone is rarely a surviving spouse, son, or daughter, nor is it likely to be the family lawyer.

Yet when the planner asks an unsophisticated estate owner whom he would designate to be an executor/trustee, the usual response is spouse or child or, occasionally, a business associate. How, then, can the planner gently suggest that a trusted family member or associate is not necessarily the ideal choice as executor? One method I have used with some success is to invite the testator to work on an IRS estate tax form. This exercise will frequently convince him that an experienced corporate or personal executor is needed—one selected on the basis of competence, objectivity, and absence of conflict of interest.

If the estate planner is capable of dealing with a terminally ill patient and his family on a sensitive yet practical level, he can render important services that will ease the burden for all. As Stephen Leimberg has put it, "By helping the client come to terms with death, and by helping him create an atmosphere in which he would be willing to die, it is easier for the client to learn to see his life in relationship with others in a clearer perspective and...(therefore) make it more meaningful" (1976).

Finally, the following maxims will prove helpful to any planner working with the terminally ill:

1. Encourage truthfulness.
2. Invite communication on all levels.
3. Allow prudence and control of one's life situation.
4. Emphasize a sense of worth.
5. Permit reality.

Surely, the terminally ill person's sense of relief in knowing his affairs have been properly ordered satisfies the requirements of these guidelines.

References

Kliman, A., and Schlesinger, E.: Counseling your dying client and his family.

SEPI. Englewood Cliffs, New Jersey, Prentice-Hall, Inc., 1979.
Kübler-Ross, E.: *On Death and Dying*. New York, Macmillan Co., 1974.
Leimberg, S.: Death sensitization for the estate planner. *CLU Journal*, April, 1976.

Chapter 28

EMOTIONAL CARE OF THE BEREAVED

Arthur M. Arkin

THE following exposition is applicable to people experiencing bereavement that results from chronic disease having afflicted the deceased, regardless of the diagnosis, i.e. death from chronic disease of all types and not exclusively from cancer. By way of preface, it must be emphasized that this chapter is based upon unsystematically structured clinical experience and psychological considerations pertaining to bereavement-associated processes. Since definitive evaluation of psychiatric therapy is well known to be a most difficult undertaking even when one has large clinic populations and high-level methodological resources at one's disposal, the clinical approaches to be described here need not be automatically considered as deficient in validity. It is my hope that experienced clinicians will recognize what is to be described as reasonable good sense.

First, I should like to pose two questions: What psychological tasks are accomplished in "healthy" grief? What psychiatric measures are available that might serve to maximize the probability of healthy grief?

In acute healthy grief, one cannot escape nor does one ordinarily wish to escape from the experience of intense pain and sadness occasioned by the loss of a person to whom one had been emotionally attached. Episodes of weeping and heartfelt sobbing are usual manifestations. It is all accepted as natural and lived through as one of life's inevitabilities. With the passage of time, the survivor liberates himself from his strong emotional ties to the deceased and learns to adapt himself to a world from which the deceased is missing. As one mourner reported in the early days of his grief, he had impulses to seek out the deceased and had the illusion of turning to a "statue of invisible silence."

This readjustment entails forming new relationships and patterns of conduct and refurbishing old ones. During the course of this sequence, one usually experiences signs and symptoms of somatic distress (sighing respiration, lack of strength, and exhaustion, gastrointestinal distress, sleep disturbances, and so forth), preoccupation with the image of the deceased, feelings of guilt toward him, inappropriate hostile reactions, and alterations in customary patterns of conduct (Lindemann, 1944). Normally, such phenomena become progressively less intense and sustained, and eventually fade.

It is impressive that the above features of grief are observable in varying degree among most bereaved even though the mourners have had an opportunity to traverse a long preterminal period of anticipatory grief. There is something about the finality of even an anticipated death that is responsible for a further increment of grief.

The family physician, religious counselor, or therapist (the helper), or whoever might be called upon to assist the grief-stricken will do well to inform himself of the details of the terminal illness and the relevant history of the family, both recent and remote, so that he may be alert to deeper psychodynamic and genetic issues. Despite the importance of confining one's explicit interventions and therapeutic comments to areas circumscribed by the *conscious and preconscious* burdens of the mourners, it is vital to guide oneself by cogent working hypotheses regarding their unconscious conflicts and to maintain close empathic contact with them.

In general, one attempts to use a supportive, empathic relationship to assist mourners in traversing their grief in the healthiest manner possible. If the deceased is survived by a family, it is reasonable, at the very least, to focus one's efforts on that family member to whom the others spontaneously turn for leadership and support. It is hoped that in this manner, therapeutic influences will filter through to those who are dependent upon him. Alternatively, should the helper sense that the others would like to join in or receive a direct request along these lines, he should not hesitate to welcome such participation in group fashion.

The following tactics have seemed clinically useful:

a. *Permitting and guiding the mourners to put into detailed words their most intimate thoughts involved in the pain, sorrow, and sense of final loss occasioned by the bereavement and to give free expression to associated affects*

An indispensable element is the verbalization of feelings of guilt toward the deceased for both recent and remote transgressions regardless, initially, of whether such guilt is appropriate. For example, one should patiently hear out the details of "if only I'd compelled him to see a doctor sooner," or "if only I had taken her on that European tour," etc.

b. *Guiding the mourner in a review of his lifelong relationship to the deceased*

The helper should be alert to important major themes, critical events, areas of appropriate guilt and of justified self-esteem for acts of devotion, thoughtfulness, authentic love, self-sacrifice, and so forth. These will enable the helper to intervene with comments and interventions aimed at promoting healthy grief. For example, if the mourner reproaches himself for a bygone episode of self-indulgence which had been partly at the expense of the deceased, it might be helpful to have on hand historical material that could demonstrate occasions when he had been thoughtful and generous toward the deceased.

c. *Providing the patient with information and understanding regarding the alterations in his emotional reactions*

Many patients feel consternation and alarm from the psychosomatic manifestations of grief and are fearful of themselves becoming ill. It is often reassuring to explain that it is natural that in grief one experiences sleep disturbances, marked heaviness of limbs, difficulty in moving about, disturbances of appetite and other gastrointestinal disturbances, headache, and so forth. Furthermore, mourners are often ashamed by their outbursts of hostility and hostile fantasies. Simple comments that this is only to be expected may be all that is necessary to bring amelioration. On the other hand, it may be useful to make some further comment to the effect that they are angry because they took the bereavement as a token of being unfairly singled out by a fate personified as cruel rather than indifferent, or that paradoxically they feel cruelly abandoned by the deceased.

d. *Assisting the patient to formulate an acceptable psychological relationship to the image of the deceased in the future*

It is important, if feasible, to help the patient acquire a future modus vivendi with his psychic representation of the deceased. For example, if the grief reaction is infused with unrealistic remorse, it is valuable to ask repeatedly whether the deceased would have wanted the survivor to live with sustained suffering. Even if the deceased had been a cruel, overly righteous individual, it may still be reasonable to raise the question as to whether he might have mellowed had he lived. Often, it is clear that the survivor, despite conscious disclaimers, believes that the deceased is not really dead but has continued living in some remote elsewhere. In such cases, it has sometimes been useful to assert the possibility that since death, the deceased may have acquired wisdom, understanding, and compassion for the plight of the mourner. In the event that the bereaved has realistic guilt toward the deceased because of some actual hostile behavior or neglect of him while alive, it may be useful to make tentative suggestions for a kind of memorial, tangible or intangible, purchased or self-created, which might provide the guilt-ridden mourner with some feeling of redemption. The important task is to attempt to arrange for a dignified and compassionate mutual farewell "within the psyche."

e. *Acting as a primer and/or programmer for some of the activities of the bereaved*

It is usually helpful to organize and direct a program for the mourner of a portion of the day's activities. This may include receiving suitable visitors, attendance at light meals, bedtimes, short walks, carrying out religious observances, and so forth. The mourner often has marked difficulty in making and executing such plans for himself and is usually grateful and benefited if someone gently guides him through such tasks.

f. *Assisting the mourner in dealing with difficult reality situations*

Such assistance includes arrangements for temporary care of children, working out legal problems, adequate financial support, shopping for food, housekeeping, and other practicalities.

g. *Arranging for formal medical and/or psychiatric measures should the need arise*

It is unwise to permit the grief-stricken to endure excessive insomnia; not only is it exhausting but tossing and turning in the early hours make the mourner vulnerable to long periods of self-torturing rumination. Prescription of bedtime sedatives for one to two weeks is often helpful. Inasmuch as stage REM sleep is thought to be of importance in the psychological mastery of stress, it is wise to prescribe an hypnotic with minimal stage REM suppression potential.

Where depression is a major and disabling feature, thought should be given to prescribing a tricyclic antidepressant. However, this should not be done hastily as it seems unwise to attempt to short-circuit the adequate traversal of grief. In general, lower dose schedules, particularly in the elderly, should be employed.

In addition, where hypochrondriacal preoccupations are prominent, thorough efforts should be made to rule out the onset of or progress of an already existing disease. One should be mindful of the demonstration that elderly people with chronic organic disease comprise a special group of patients possessing a higher degree of post-bereavement vulnerability (Wiener et al., 1975).

Finally, certain morbid reactions may be observed and should occasion a consultation with a specialist who is informed about grief and its pathological forms. The three most common forms of pathological grief are—

1. Delayed grief with variable degree of expression at some subsequent date
2. Inhibited grief with minimal or absent indications of "conventional" mourning but with the onset of psychosomatic symptoms and behavior patterns that may be understood as substitutes for or equivalents of the inhibited grief
3. Prolonged and over-intense grief (chronic grief) often with intense guilt and self-reproach. Other more subtle variants and additional components are described in the specialized literature (Parkes, 1965)

h. *Contraindicated interventions*
   1. Psychological interpretation of key defenses against highly charged, warded off, unconscious mental content
   2. Excessive solicitude and overprotection of the patient

In general, the baseline attitude of the helper, from which appropriate departures may be made, should be one of compassionate but temperate empathic concern, avoiding sentimentality and too much identification. The therapist should recognize the full extent of the emotional loss but, nevertheless, gently convey to the patient, after subsidence of the acute, initial, intense phase of grief, that it is the normal, expected course that he recover like anyone else, that life must go on, and that the mourner possesses the required inner strength to make a new life or to carry on. The helper should make it clear that he would like to make himself available for subsequent sessions on an irregular ad lib basis at a frequency of once weekly or less. Assistance should be offered in making future plans of all types, including possible appropriate changes in occupation, residence, social life, and so on.

Normally, acute grief lasts one or two months and gradually subsides and recedes by about six months. Reactivation may occur with the anniversary of the death or stimulation of stressful memories involving the deceased. The plans of the helper should take these time factors into account.

References

Lindemann, E.: Symptomatology and management of acute grief. *American Journal of Psychiatry, 101*:141-148, 1944.

Parkes, C.M.: Bereavement and mental illness. *British Journal of Medical Psychology, 38*:1-26, 1965.

Wiener, A., Gerber, I., Battin, D., and Arkin, A.: The process and phenomenology of bereavement. In B. Schoenberg et al.: *Bereavement: Its Psychosocial Aspects.* New York, Columbia University Press, 1975.

Chapter 29

VARIANTS OF PATHOLOGICAL BEREAVEMENT

GEORGE KRUPP AND CAROL LANDAU

THE experience of loss by death is an expectable but always shocking life crisis; it intrudes itself into the life of the survivor, challenging ordinary coping responses and setting off a process of adaptation that begins with denial and ends in eventual readaptation to life without the lost one. Many societies have cultural rituals to aid in the readaptation process so that mourners are helped to assimilate the loss; however, in our twentieth-century American society, with its stress on avoidance and denial of death, pathologic grief responses are unwittingly promoted.

Health professionals often see people exhibiting bereavement reactions and have difficulty distinguishing normal grieving from pathological responses. Pathology expresses itself on a continuum between those whose defenses allow a normal adaptation and those on the other extreme who develop outright neurotic responses or psychosomatic or psychotic symptoms. This paper will discuss the process and components of normal grieving contrasted with pathologic responses; it will suggest aspects of our culture that predispose toward pathologic bereavement; and then, more specifically, it will discuss some factors in the circumstances of the loss—the person and the situation—that may also predispose to pathology.

The components of normal grieving are both conscious and unconscious and are the organism's way of biologically attempting to assimilate the loss. The first stage is the attempt to recapture the lost object (protest and denial). Then, responding to the futility of this activity, there is a stage of despair and disorganization. The third stage is to finally relinquish the attempt to regain the lost one (reorganization and hope) and to develop new adaptations to living.

Protest and Denial

The first realization of a death results in shock and numbness and often anger and guilt, which may last a short or long time but which constitute a powerful defense enabling the mourner to assimilate the reality of the loss gradually. The "urge to recover the lost object," as described by Bowlby (1961), is expressed in the weeping and anger reminiscent of infant attempts to summon the mother. In this phase, dreams and hallucinations of the dead person may be experienced.

Despair and Disorganization

As the loss is experienced, denied, and reexperienced, a second phase develops: despair and disorganization, marked by depression, agitation, anxiety, and feelings of emptiness. Disorganization begins within hours of the death and reaches its height within a few days or weeks, but it can continue even longer. Isolation of affect, avoidance of others, and obsessive preoccupations are some of the defenses employed during this period.

Reorganization and Hope

"Reality passes its verdict, in that the object no longer exists — upon each single one of the memories and hopes through which the libido was attached to the lost object; and the ego, confronted as it were, over a decision whether it will share this fate, is persuaded by the sum of its narcissistic satisfactions in being alive, to sever its attachment to the nonexistent object." This description by Freud (1917) of the *work of mourning* indicates that the bereaved chooses to extricate the energy and love felt first toward the lost one, to redirect it toward the introject of the loved one, and then to transfer the energy back toward other people. This period may take months and in the normal person usually begins in one to two months. However, the process may not be complete for years, i.e. the forming of new relationships and the development of new roles in life without the lost one. Studies show that even after many, many months following an acute loss, a significant percentage of people remain depressed. While many continue to mourn, a few are suicidal (Greenblatt, 1978).

There are important components of grief that reflect the individual's attempt to deal with unconscious conflicts, but they do not constitute pathologic responses unless they result in the inability of the mourner to give up attempts to recover the lost person. Pathologic bereavement occurs when the individual remains fixed in the first two stages of protest and disorganization.

What are the components of mourning, i.e. the emotional and physical reactions occurring throughout the phases of mourning?

1. *Somatic feelings* are universal, especially in the earliest phases. They include exhaustion, increased tendency to sighing, loss of appetite, a feeling of emptiness in the stomach, weeping, insomnia, appearance of woodenness, restlessness, increase in irritability, and fear. These symptoms come and go, and according to Parkes (1972) they could be viewed as an alarm reaction resulting from heightened stimulation of the sympathetic nervous system. Symptoms of the deceased that represent internalization of the lost one may also be present (Krupp, 1965).

2. A universal and powerful feeling is one of *anger*, often unconscious and seemingly irrational. This ties up with previous negative feelings toward the deceased, and now new, more insistent anger emerges toward the dead one for the act of abandonment. With such hostility present, it invariably has to be tied in with guilt. Sometimes the anger is displaced onto third parties: God, the hospital, nurse, relative, or doctor. The anger accompanying such powerful feelings of loss has biological roots. Consider an elephant in the jungle who is separated from her calf. The mother elephant reacts with great anxiety and anger and goes crashing through the jungle looking for her lost baby.

Bowlby (1963) has linked the relationship of grief in infancy and mourning in animals to adult bereavement. He points out that the adaptive function of hostility in infants and animals is an attempt to recover the lost love object and to ensure no future loss. He cites examples of dogs that after losing a master became disobedient, delinquent, and savage.

Expressions of hostility are seen in preliterate society. "In many tribes special precautions are taken against violent outbursts verging on homicidal attacks, on the part of the mourners" (Devereux, 1942). Self-inflicted wounds, so common in primitive society, and actual and symbolic eating of the dead may be partially understood in this context. In some societies, the funeral customs express "strong sanctions against violence" (Southall, 1960), and any hostile feelings present are focused on absent people thought to have used supernatural means to cause the death. Durkheim (1915) writes of the anger mixed in with the ceremonies. Quarrels are provoked, combats are organized, tortures are self-inflicted. "They also throw themselves on the ground, and mutually beat and tear each other."*

Feelings of anger are also experienced toward the dead person. These are often below conscious awareness. The mourner is angry at the person who caused his painful state, which often creates feelings of remorse and guilt.

3. *Guilt.* Sometimes guilt can lead to idealization of the deceased (retroactive falsification) and may represent an attempt at restitution and a defense against the pain. The guilt feelings may be related to the hostility previously felt. The death reactivates any ambivalence that was present, and if this was strong, the result is self-reproach. There is also guilt because of the lack of ability to undo previous negative attitudes and behavior toward the lost one. Unconsciously, the mourner may feel that he has brought about the death by his wish. At times, the bereaved may even have fantasies that the dead person may seek revenge and kill him.†

These feelings have their roots in infantile feelings of omnipotence. As children well into the latency period, we all have powerful feelings of importance, having experienced ourselves via the solicitude of nurturers as the center of the world. Fantasies during this period seem very powerful, and children often fear that their thoughts have the power to affect events. Anxiety over fears about death are reduced by the thought that "if one is good, dying may be warded off or the effects of dying reversed." Piaget (1954) points out that in the period of concrete operations, children believe death is a violent force controllable by acts of good. He tells the story recalled by Mlle. Ve, told by Flourney regarding a child's magical idea that his own action or thought can influence events:

> One of the most distant memories relates to my mother. She was very ill and had been in bed several weeks and a servant had told me she would die in a few days. I must have been about four or five years old. My most treasured possession was a little, brown, wooden horse, covered with "real hair." ... A curious thought came into my head. I must give up my horse

---

*It is very helpful in working with mourners for them to learn that their anger is normal and also has a biological foundation. This knowledge aids in relieving guilt and lessening the anger.

†In preliterate societies, large stones were frequently placed on the grave to prevent the dead one from returning, and it is believed that this is the origin of the tombstone.

in order to make my mother better. It was more than I could do at once and cost me the greatest pain. I started by throwing the saddle and bridle into the fire, thinking that "when it's very ugly I shall be able to keep it." I can't remember exactly what happened. But I know that in the greatest distress, I ended by smashing my horse to bits and that on seeing my mother up a few days later, I was convinced that it was my sacrifice that had mysteriously cured her and this conviction lasted for a long while.

The feelings of guilt are often holdovers from these childhood conceptions of infantile omnipotence. Rochlin (1965) states that what is remarkable is not that children arrive at adult concepts of death, but how tenaciously throughout life adults readily revert to the child's beliefs. We carry these defenses throughout life — the belief in the omnipotence of wishes and the power of hope, the imperishable egocentricity, the sense of helplessness and dependency and the dread of abandonment.

Another component of guilt may be the survivor response. There is a natural relief that the self is intact, and feelings of unconscious triumph may also increase the guilt. Guilt likewise may be generated by the awareness of satisfying secondary gains from the death. One's wish for concern and attention from others is gratified at the price of the death, another unconscious source of inner conflict.

4. *Feelings of helplessness* are usually present because of an inability to do anything about the loss and because of awareness that continuing future life will be without the presence of the partner.

5. *Anxiety*, also biological, is usually present, and may be a response due to the fear of being alone and helpless. Fear of one's own death may also cause anxiety. The mourner may relive the infantile terror that his hate and lack of love have brought on the loss. Occasionally, in the case of the loss of a parent, fear of a close incestuous involvement with the other parent may occur.

6. *Old conflicts* are apt to reappear. The loss may stir up past loss reactions and may also exacerbate incompleted resolutions of sibling and oedipal conflicts and problems of dependence or independence. Analytically, the reaction to any separation or loss throughout life may be viewed as reactivation of the infantile depressive position that occurred at the time of early separations.

The reactivation of old conflicts could have an adaptive function for the mourner. At the time of condolence calls, it is common to hear the friends or family of the primary mourners recall their own former losses; when they are with the actively grieving person, all find thoughts of other losses, other expressions of grief, or other comforting experiences. These recollections are important and serve an adaptive function in the mourning process. Much as small children attempt to master conflict situations by going over them repeatedly in play, so the mourner by going over past losses and death experiences attempts to deal emotionally with the unthinkable loss.

7. *Denial*, a common emotion, is usually an integral component of the initial reaction to most important losses. It often remains difficult to face reality even long afterward. The mourner may continue behavior as if the dead one were still alive, and the denial may surface when the pain is too great to bear.

8. *Absence of emotion* is closely related to denial and in the earlier period of the mourning process may be regarded as quite normal. It may be a postponement of the painful "work of mourning" until the reality becomes unavoidable. Here again, absence of emotion may provide help in lessening the shock and grief.

A bereaved person sometimes feels liberated from the influence of the lost one. There have been cases of schizophrenia, where there was excessive involvement with parents, which go into a state of remission shortly after the death of the patient's parent.

9. *Relief* is another feeling, especially when there was a long and painful illness preceding the death. The mourner feels relieved that the loved one no longer is in pain or that the burden of caring for the dying has been lifted. The bereaved may also experience relief from the anxiety of the anticipated death.

It seems clear from this review that grief and mourning are not simple emotions. "The pain of loss and its attendant yearning for a deceased loved one are merely the more familiar external facets of a highly complex reaction. In its primary sense, grief over death is fettered anger—anger at the injustice done to the self—not only through the actual loss, but through the dependence, the loneliness and the *inconvenience* it may bring" (Krupp, 1972).

Before discussing pathology, it is important to emphasize that our American culture is very conducive to production of pathological mourning. It may be illustrated by comparing the way our culture deals with the universal problems that occur in a death with the way preliterate societies deal with these same problems (Krupp and Kligfeld, 1962).

What are these universal problems that every society deals with? Cultural evaluation of mourning rituals indicates that an individual's bereavement is conditioned not only by his early reaction to loss and biological adaptive mechanisms but also by the specific institutionalized ways provided by the culture for dealing with the loss. The problems in bereavement are universal: (1) how to explain death; (2) loathing of the corpse — problems of disposal; (3) fear of cause of death, the dead one — the role of hostility and projection; (4) desire for continued interaction with the lost one being transformed into a quest for immortality; and (5) the impact of death on the community and how it reintegrates itself.

In preliterate societies, pathological bereavement is less common because of (1) proximity to natural processes; (2) absence of intense involvement and availability of substitute resources; (3) prescribed rituals that aid in working through loss; and (4) persistent belief that the person is not really lost but that there is merely a change in communication.

Why then is our American culture conducive to pathological bereavement?

Many things in our culture conspire to remove death from our minds and even our feelings. Television, movies, and even the expression of our mores put emphasis on youth and how to preserve it. Death is then threatening and difficult to handle; so it is made remote. The elderly and sick are rarely kept at home. They are removed from the family so as not to remind us of death. Death has become forbidding, repugnant, and mysterious. The bereaved is expected to control his emotions and make his state less noticeable. The funeral home, the flowers, the music, and even the makeup on the deceased are all ways to deny death. Friends look at the corpse and describe it as so "life like." Self-control is frequently rewarded and praised.

Our emphasis on the individual is shown in the avoidance of rituals for mourning. Aside from the rites of funeral chapel, church, or synagogues, and the retention of some Old World forms of communal involvement in the family's loss, the individual is largely left alone to adjust to all the changes in status and role.

Preliterate cultures, however, did not put so much emphasis on the importance of the individual. When one died, others took over his role and status. There, they had broader relationships with more people and less focus on self. In contrast, our society permits greater freedom of choice of love objects and emphasis on the uniqueness of the individual. The greater range for identification and greater awareness of self promote isolation. There are fewer people to relate to and a more intimate relationship develops among these.

This intimacy to fewer people is one of the main characteristics that makes bereavement so personally significant and anxiety-producing in our culture. Another aspect is the long childhood dependency on parents not seen in preliterate cultures.

We also have the idea, in our highly scientific and technological society, that there are and should be answers for everything. Faced with death, especially when the circumstances do not seem to be in the expectable course of events, we have more difficulty in meeting the reality than do societies that are not so omnipotent in their needs for mastery.

We have reviewed the components of normal mourning and some aspects of our twentieth-century American culture that promote poor adaptation to death. The remainder of this chapter will concern itself with pathologic grief and some of the determinant factors that seem to dispose some people to respond maladaptively.

Inability to rearrange the threads of one's life in one or many ways is evidence of a pathological grief response. How does this pathology evidence itself? What are the signs and symptoms of a pathologic mourning response? "Normal behavior is essentially rational, adaptive, flexible, and conscious. In normal bereavement, therefore, there is ultimately a reorganization of behavior. Behavior which is focused on the lost object and based on the desire to achieve reunion is irrational and nonadaptive. It is gradually discarded" (Krupp, 1972).

Pathological Bereavement

1. If any of the components of mourning outlined earlier are *excessively intense*, one may consider that to be maladaptive. This is a difficult differentiation unless the behavior is extreme. It may be accompanied by nightmares, outbursts of fear and anger, and strong feelings that the mourner has no right to be alive. Intense guilt gives rise to the conviction that the mourner must be punished, that he must make amends by dying, too. This guilt may even lead to sui-

cide. Shakespeare's character Hamlet embodies a bereavement containing elements of ambivalence, oedipal guilt, murder, psychosis, and suicide.

2. One of the most common pathological mourning reactions is the *prolonged* one in which the bereavement reaction becomes chronic and leads to a true depression.

3. Anxiety regarding ambivalent unconscious responses can also surface as an *absence of mourning*. This response is frequently seen in adolescents who have had a primary loss. They themselves are struggling with the life task of adjusting to the loss of childhood, which is being wrenched from them. The reality of death can be unbearably anxiety-provoking if it occurs during this adolescent period, and powerful denial can result in the avoidance of mourning, a danger signal suggesting maladaptive response. If the denial is not overcome or if the mourner does not respond to the loss at all, then it must be regarded as pathological.

Helene Deutsch observes (1937), "First, that the death of a beloved person must produce reactive expression of feeling in the normal course of events; second, that omission of such reactive responses is to be considered just as much a variation from the normal as excess in time or intensity and, third, that unmanifested grief will be found expressed to the full in some way or other."

4. The development of *physical illness* is another expression of pathologic bereavement. It has been suggested that ulcerative colitis and rheumatoid or osteoarthritis are often somatic sequelae of bereavement and that coronary thrombosis, blood cancers, and cancer of the uterus may be aggravated (Parkes, 1972; Epstein et al., 1975). Lynch (1978) has pointed out that social isolation, sudden loss of love, death or absence of parents in early childhood, and lack of human companionship can be contributors to premature death from a variety of medical reasons.

Studies have shown that widows under the age of sixty reflected with statistical significance more health deterioration than married women in the control group (Epstein et al., 1975).

5. *Psychiatric Illness*: Often a bereavement will exacerbate a preexisting but perhaps dormant psychotic predisposition, which may or may not have surfaced previously. Parkes (1972) studied 3,245 patients admitted to a psychiatric unit over a two-year period and discovered that 194 developed illness within six months of a

death of a spouse or parents (6 percent). Care needs to be taken to understand such symptoms as occasional hallucinations and obsessive preoccupation with the deceased as being within the normal boundaries of grieving, though they are frightening to the bereaved and often lead them to fear they are going crazy. True psychotic responses are prolonged and intense and reflect distortions of reality, leading to maladaptive behaviors such as self-isolation, belligerence, immobilizing depressions, and hypochondriacal preoccupations.

6. Another pathological reaction occurs when a child loses a loved one and develops some *arrested psychosocial development*. This is very common and not fully recognized by physicians. Studies of Blueck, Johnson et al., as noted in Epstein et al. (1975), suggest links between loss in childhood and antisocial behavior, increases in violence, reduced academic achievement, and social withdrawal. The depth of the loss may not fully manifest itself until the child becomes a parent. At that time, the loss is relived, and the individual tries to protect his child from the same hurt.

7. *Somatic symptoms of the lost person*. This pathological identification permits the mourner to retain the dead one in fantasy, as if he were alive. This reaction is a gain in one sense but also represents guilt and punishment. The unconscious dynamics behind these symptoms are illustrated by the patient who experiences heart symptoms following a father's death by heart attack. These conversion reactions representing unconscious gain (bringing back the lost one) are also a punishment. It is, in its way, a variation of the familiar theme of an eye for an eye, a tooth for a tooth. Justice results when the survivor punishes himself with the same kind of suffering that had been endured by the dying.

8. *Personality identifications in the mourner, who adopts mannerisms, traits, and characteristics of the loved one*. These represent unconscious attempts to bring back the person and often, paradoxically, consist of behavior that the mourner disliked. Identification in mourning is not simply the haphazard adoption of a loved person's traits. It depends on such factors as the previous relationships, the ambivalence,* the area of conflict, the content of what is introjected, the effects, needs, and drives involved and the purpose for which identification is util-

---

*"A stable adjustment to another's death involves assimilating both the loved and hated elements of his personality. As a consequence, the bereaved must experience some safe hate, some self hate, some self-accusation, some guilt" (Pincus, 1974).

ized.

Why, for instance, is a particular trait selected for identification? At any given time, the personality trait or symptom selected for identification may serve a particular purpose. For example, one patient, a physician's daughter, developed her mother's terminal symptoms when, during periods of stress, she desired her father's support and interest. By this device, she could, despite her antagonism toward her father, allow herself to approach him. Her knowledge that he had been particularly solicitous toward her mother in her final illness unconsciously reinforced the symptoms.

Identification may occur when the death wish is strongest, as in the case of a son, who, while having sexual relations with a woman (unconsciously his mother), develops his father's heart symptoms. Yet when this same son needs father during stress, the identification takes on a different form.

Identification seems more apt to occur in mourners who had intense relationships with the deceased person but may be present following illness without death. It occurred in one patient who "looked down at my hands and saw my mother's" at a time when she was making desperate attempts to reduce an involvement with her healthy mother.

9. *Loneliness of the bereaved.* Loneliness may be one of the greatest problems of the widowed. A widow who has her own profession and interests, independent of her husband, is in a more favorable position. The more involvement in the husband–wife relationship, the more disorganized the bereaved is apt to become.

As health professionals begin to clarify what appear to be normal bereavement responses contrasted with pathologic bereavement, focus begins more toward evaluation of determinant factors predisposing to poor bereavement response. Several significant areas are potential predictors of response:

1. *The nature of the loss incurred* may be predictive of the bereavement response. The suddenness, degree of preparedness of the mourner, circumstances of the death, and perception of the preventability or inevitability of the death all may affect the adaptation process. An interesting study of sixty-eight widows and widowers by Parkes (1975) suggested that poor bereavement outcome correlated highly with short terminal illness with little warning of the death. However, conflicting studies also exist and suggest that protracted

death, associated with severe suffering and disfigurement, tended to aggravate whatever ambivalences existed in the relationship and were predictors of unfavorable outcome (Epstein et al., 1975). It has been suggested that there is a correlation of poor response between the centrality of the lost person in the life of the mourner and the mourner's perception of the preventability of death (Bugen, 1977).

If one postulates that some of the guilt response experienced by survivors rests with infantile omnipotent fantasies, then the degree to which one imagines he could have prevented the death would have an effect on the response to the loss.

2. *The preexisting relationship* between the lost person and the bereaved can be predictive of possibly poor bereavement response if the relationship was highly ambivalent and particularly if that ambivalence needs to be heavily denied by the mourner (Peretz, 1970). The Parkes study (1975) found a high correlation between crises within the marital relationship and poor response. An interesting finding in this study was that people who reflected high ambivalence in the marital relationship were significantly more likely to have lost a mother by illness or to have had parents who were separated or divorced. Other studies have suggested that poor interpersonal relationships with the person's mother or with the family of the deceased are also predictive of poor response (Epstein, 1975).

Excessive dependence in a relationship is also predictive of potential poor outcome. This relates to the point made earlier in this paper regarding the cultural focus on intense but few significant relationships. If the lost person was experienced not as a separate person but as an extension of the self, the loss will be experienced as a loss within the self—a narcissistic injury—and grieving will be intense and prolonged. Such people often have difficulty in accepting the fact of a loss and show a high degree of yearning over a long period (Parkes, 1975). Another aspect of the relationship between the deceased and the griever relates to the importance that the lost one represented in the social system and is another kind of predictor of outcome.

3. Situational stressors can be predictive of poor response; if the loss is followed by lowering of the socioeconomic status of survivors, a poor grief response often occurs (Lindemann, 1944). The 1975 Parkes study also showed a statistically significant correlation between low socioeconomic status and poor outcome, especially where

there were large numbers of children at home. This seems to corroborate other studies suggesting that widows under forty-five with dependent children have difficulty adapting to their new life (Maddison, 1967). Not only are they less likely to be able to move freely into the social scene because of financial lack and need to be available to the children, but also they are less likely to have opportunity to grieve openly and directly themselves, because focus will be on the needs of the youngsters. Health care providers and social planners, by being sensitized, may address themselves to the special needs of these women at the time of bereavement.

A person experiencing additional crises, such as change of job or home, at the same time as a bereavement, may have a poor grief outcome, especially if handling of the secondary crises aborts the grieving process. Volkan (1970) makes an important contribution to our understanding when he describes grieving as being like an "insurance against later pathology." When circumstances conspire to suppress the grieving process, one can expect later maladaptive responses.

4. *Absence or poor quality of support systems* available to the bereaved has an effect on the bereavement response. The lack of extended family systems in our society places inordinate pressure on the nuclear family in responding to loss. The availability of others during all the phases can be significantly helpful but only if the input from those significant others permits expressions of grief. Maddison's study (1967) of bereaved widows suggested that widows dissatisfied with help available to them during the crisis often had a poor outcome, as well as preexisting mental illness. Persons who had prior history of severe reaction to death of another family member may be likely to repeat the response (Epstein et al., 1975).

5. *Losses* may revive infantile separation anxieties. People who have had severe early deprivations or difficulty handling separations, minor as well as major, may be expected to have difficulty assimilating a loss by death (Barlow, 1974).

Clayton (1978) has conducted a bereavement study not only considering pathology in terms of frequency of symptoms but also considering their course. In contrast to findings that show a higher percent of pathological grief, she states, "The 16 percent of the subjects who continued to be troubled by low mood, and many symptoms, were found more likely to have had a preexisting psychiatric illness or a problem such as alcoholism."

In conclusion, there is no norm for mourning or adaptation, nor is there any time limit for either. Many make apparently successful resolutions; then, in special situations, such as an anniversary or illness, there may be a brief regression. The criterion for a pathological state is that the mourner is unable to cope with life. Only when the lost person has been internalized with a constructive identification has an adjustment to a new life been made.

Summary

Individuals exhibiting pathological bereavement reactions appear to be in the *middle portion* of a continuum between those who are on the one end, representing so-called normal grief reactions with good resolutions, and those on the other end of the spectrum, who develop outright neuroses, psychosomatic symptoms, and conversion symptoms that are directly related to the known loss. Pathological reactions to the loss of a loved one are probably more common than is recognized by the medical profession, including psychiatrists and other mental health personnel.

To cope with the emotional problems following death, man has developed culturally prescribed rituals. The function of the funeral rite is twofold: to maintain the integrity of the community and to force the individual to work through the loss. Mourning rituals express the ambivalence of the individual and society toward the deceased and protect against projected hostility. The permanence of the loss is denied and minimized as being only a change in communication.

In preliterate societies, pathological bereavement is less common because of (a) proximity to natural resources, (b) absence of intense involvement and availability of substitute resources, and (c) prescribed rituals that aid in working through the loss.

All these factors are less significant in our society. Death has become frightening, mysterious, and repugnant, and yet the bereaved is often supposed to behave well. Death has become alien and more frightening; hence the bereavement reaction is severe, frequently producing the pathological states.

Pathological mourning reactions include (1) excessively intense reactions, (2) prolonged mourning, (3) absence of mourning,

(4) development of physical illness, (5) production of psychiatric illness, and (6) arrested psychosocial development, (7) somatic symptoms of the lost person, and (8) personality identifications in the mourner.

Factors predictive of poor outcome include (1) nature of loss—suddenness, prolonged suffering, concepts of inevitability; (2) preexisting relationship—ambivalence denied, excessive dependency; (3) situational stressors—socioeconomic situations, widows with young children, additional crises in addition to death; (4) absence of support systems or poor quality of support systems; and (5) former severe response to loss.

References

Barlow, J.M.: Loss and mourning: Some implications for psychotherapy. *Journal of Tennessee Medical Association,* 67:834-836, 1974.

Bowlby, J.: Processes of mourning. *International Journal of Psychoanalysis,* 42:317-340, 1961.

Bowlby, J.M.: Pathological mourning and childhood mourning. *Journal of American Psychoanalytic Association,* 11:3, 1963.

Bugen, L.A.: Human grief: A model for prediction and intervention. *American Journal of Orthopsychiatry,* 47 (April):2, 1977.

Clayton, P.J.: Talk at 68th Meeting of the American Psychopathological Association, 1978.

Deutsch, H.: Absence of grief. *Psychoanalytic Quarterly,* 6:12-22, 1937.

Devereux, G.: Primitive psychiatry: Funeral suicide and the Mohave social structure. *Bulletin of the History of Medicine,* 1:522-542, 1942.

Durkheim, E.: *The Elementary Forms of the Religious Life.* London, Allen and Unwin, 1915.

Epstein, G., Weitz, L., et al.: Research on bereavement: A selective critical review. *Comprehensive Psychiatry,* 16, 1975.

Freud, S.: Mourning and melancholia. *Collected Papers, Volume 4.* New York, Basic Books, 1959.

Greenblatt, M.: The grieving spouse. *American Journal of Psychiatry,* 135:1, 1978.

Krupp, G.: Identification as a defense against anxiety in coping with loss. *International Journal of Psychoanalysis,* 46 (July):303-314, 1965.

Krupp, G.: Maladaptive reactions to the death of a family member. *Social Casework,* 53 (July):425-434, 1972.

Krupp, G., and Kligfeld, B.: The bereavement reactions: A cross-cultural evaluation. *Journal of Religion and Health,* 1:222-246, 1962.

Lindemann, E.: Symptomatology and management of acute grief. *American Journal of Psychiatry,* 101:141-148, 1944.

Lynch, J.J.: *The Broken Heart: The Medical Consequences of Loneliness in America.* New York, Basic Books, 1978.

Maddison, D.: Factors affecting the outcome of conjugal bereavement. *British Journal of Psychiatry, 113*:1057-1067, 1967.

Parkes, C.M.: *Bereavement: Studies of Grief in Adult Life.* New York, International Universities Press, 1972.

Parkes, C.M.: Unexpected and untimely bereavement: A statistical study of young Boston widows and widowers. In Schoenberg, B., et al.: *Bereavement: Its Psychosocial Aspects.* New York, Columbia University Press, 1975.

Peretz, D.: Reactions to loss. In Schoenberg, B., et al.: *Loss and Grief: Psychological Management in Medical Practice.* New York, Columbia University Press, 1970.

Piaget, J.: *The Construction of Reality in the Child.* New York, Basic Books, 1954.

Pincus, L.: *Death and the Family: The Importance of Mourning.* New York, Pantheon Books, 1974.

Rochlin, G.: *Griefs and Discontents: The Forces of Change.* Boston, Little, Brown and Co., 1965.

Southall, A.W.: *Homicide and Suicide Among the Alur: African Homicide and Suicide.* Princeton University Press, 1960.

Volkan, V.: Typical findings in pathological grief. *Psychoanalytic Quarterly, 44*:2, 1970.

Chapter 30

A CONFIDENTIAL FAMILY FINANCIAL CHECKLIST

EDWIN NADEL AND JOHN J. PARKER

The facts in this checklist will help the patient, his advisors and family members coordinate affairs of financial concern. It has been broken down into 15 different sections dealing with personal data, income requirements, various questions, disability insurance, life insurance details, other assets, storage of papers, investment plans, estate objectives, taxes, distribution considerations, discussions about maturing trusts and anticipating inheritances, other pertinent data, and a checklist for other documents needed for analysis.

I

Date _____

Name _____	Company _____
Residence Address _____	Business Address _____
Phone _____ Years there _____	Phone _____ Years there _____
Date of Marriage _____	Nature of Business _____ Title _____

FAMILY DATA

Name	Relationship	Birth Date	Birth Place	M or S	Health*	S.S. No.

*Physician

Family Information _____ Stepchildren — Adopted _____

Earning Ability of all (Use separate sheet if necessary) _____

Other Dependents — Parents, In-laws, etc. _____ Extent of Support _____

Previous Marriage _____ Divorce _____ Separation Agreement _____ Date _____

HOME OWNERSHIP

1. Mortgage Date _____ Amount _____ Interest _____% Term ____

   Monthly charges _____ Unpaid balance _____ Prepayment privilege _____

2. Do you wish home free and clear? _____ Or extra monthly payments? _____

3. Any Home improvements: _____

4. Can you make a list of costs, dates, and descriptions? _____
   _____
   _____

II
FAMILY CASH AND INCOME REQUIREMENTS

A. Monthly Income   C. Settlement Funds

1. Dependency period $ _____   1. Current expenses $ _____

2. Readjustment for ____ yrs. _____   2. Obligations   _____

3. Life Income   _____   3. Final expenses   _____

   (Outside income $ _____)   4. Taxes: a) Income   _____
                                                      (quarterly
                                                      estimate)
                                                   b) Property   _____
                                                   c) Death   _____

A Confidential Family Financial Checklist

B. Special Cash Needs	D. Special Income Needs
1. Mortgage $ _____	1. Parents? _____ _____
2. Emergency fund _____	2. _____ _____
3. Educational fund _____	3. _____ _____
4. Any litigation? _____	
5. Any special bequest? _____	
6. Charity _____	
7. _____ _____	

III
QUESTIONS

1. What is the managerial and business ability of spouse? _____
2. What is the managerial and business ability of children? _____
3. What is their business experience? _____
4. Can spouse or other family members draw income from business at death of principal? _____
5. What Group Insurance does your company offer? _____
6. Does your company have a $5,000.00 tax-free death benefit? _____
7. Does your company have a pension or profit-sharing plan? _____
   What are your benefits if you:
         Terminate: _____   Become Disabled: _____
         Die: _____
         Can Life Insurance be added to the plan? _____
8. Are you able to borrow? _____
   _____ (Discuss in Detail.)
9. Burial arrangements? _____
10. Obituary? _____
11. Do you own any Flower Bonds? _____
12. Do you have Annuity Payments? _____ Will they continue to others? _____

IV
YOUR CAREER-JOB-BUSINESS

Describe: _____

_____

Should you change jobs? _____

Income: _____ Benefits: _____

V
DISABILITY INCOME

1. Total Income required during disability? _____

2. Professional Overhead Expense or Business Overhead Expense:

Rent	$ ____	Periodicals	$ ____	Elec., Oil, Gas, etc.	$ ____
Property Taxes	____	Maintenance Service	____	Dues:	____
Property Ins. Prem.	____	Equipment Depreciation	____	Other Fixed Expense	____
Property Mtge. Int.	____	Liability Insurance Premiums	____		
Employees' Salaries	____				
Sub-Total	$ ____	Sub-Total	$ ____	TOTAL	$ ____

3. Are you covered by a State Disability Program? _____
4. a) Major Medical Plan? _____ b) Hospitalization? _____
   c) Will company pay medical bills? _____ d) Can Major Medical be continued by family? _____
5. How long secy./nurse/or key employee working for you? _____
6. To what societies do you belong? _____
7. Termination clause in lease? _____
8. Any Disability Buy and Sell Agreements? _____
9. What is the company's policy with respect to paying executives who become disabled permanently or for a long period of time? _____
10. Where are disability insurance policies stored? _____

VI
LIFE INSURANCE DETAILS

Where are insurance policies stored? _____ Who owns them? _____

Are there any loans? _____ Are they insured? _____

What are you doing with your dividends? _____ Any with company? _____

What are you doing with your paid-up additions? _____

Do you have your last premium notices? _____

Do you have any group insurance? _____

Is there insurance on your wife or children? _____ Why? _____

                                                                                                                  Why Not? _____

Is your life insurance beneficiary the same as your will? _____

      Has this been checked? _____

What are your insurance objectives? _____

Any Group Creditors Insurance? _____

      Any Convertible Decreasing Term? _____

Should Business Insurance become personal insurance? _____

Purchase Options? _____ Family Agreements? _____

VII

	Date Acq.	Cost Values	Situs State	Gross Values			Loans**	Income	Hard to Sell***	Liquid
				Husb.	Wife	Joint*				
Real Estate										
Savings Acct's										
Checking Acct's										
Gov't Bonds										
Mutual Funds										
Stocks										
Bonds										
Personal Effects										
Special Equip, etc. Art-Antiques										
Notes										
Mortgages										
Patents & Royalties										
Life Ins. Face Amount										
Ins. Cash Values Other Lives										
Pension/Profit-Sharing										
Interest in Trusts										
Deferred Comp. Stock Option										
Vested Interests										
Business Int.										
Power of Appointments										
Children's Assets (Owned by H. or W.)										
Total										
Any Loans Separate H.W. Joint										
Net Assets at Death										

*Percentage of Gift
**Insured
**Indicate Husband, Wife or Joint
*** Should assets be sold NOW — Discuss

A Confidential Family Financial Checklist 229

VIII
STORAGE OF IMPORTANT PAPERS OR DOCUMENTS

1. Assets on Previous Page _____   8. Trust Instrument _____
2. Wills _____   9. Children's Bankbooks _____
3. Marriage Certificate _____   10. Travelers Checks _____
4. Birth Certificate _____   11. Stamp Collection _____
5. Divorce Decree _____   12. Coin Collection _____
6. Tax Returns _____   13. Agreements _____
7. Discharge Papers _____   14. _____

IX
INVESTMENT PLANS

1. Investment Plans _____ Surplus for Investment _____
2. Special program for children? _____
3. Investment ability of wife? _____

X
ESTATE OBJECTIVES

_____

_____

XI
TAXES

Income Tax paid last year — State $ _____ Federal $ _____ City $ _____

Please furnish copies of last year's tax returns.

XII
DISTRIBUTION CONSIDERATIONS

1. Special Family needs:
2. Charitable bequests:

XII
DISTRIBUTION CONSIDERATIONS (con't)

3. Trusts (Describe):   Past:

   Contemplated:

4. Should current assets of children be used for education or living expenses?
5. Disposition of Business Interests (Retention or Sale)

6. Gifts: Past: To Whom   When   Present or Future Value   Return Submitted   Total Exemp. Used

   Contemplated:

XIII
MATURING TRUSTS, ANTICIPATED INHERITANCES, LEGACIES

1. Self:
2. Other Family Members:
3. Review estate plan of other family members:

XIV
PERTINENT DATA   VERIFY RECORDS

1. Social Security Coverage? _____ No. _____ Since _____
2. Veteran? _____ Entered _____ Discharged _____ GI No. _____
   Service Connected Disability? _____ Reason _____ Claim No. _____
3. Will? _____ Date: _____ State: _____ Executor: _____
4. Spouse's Will? _____ Date: _____ State: _____ Executor: _____
5. Guardian: _____
6. Advisors: Please provide full name, mailing address, and telephone
   (Use separate sheet)

   Attorneys: _____   Accountant: _____

   Insurance Advisor: _____

A Confidential Family Financial Checklist 231

Advisors (con't)

Life Insurance Advisor: _____

Investment Advisor: _____

Trust Officer: _____

Psychiatrist: _____

Clergy—Friends _____

Have you spoken with these Advisors? Have you discussed fees?
Paid fees? _____ How much will the fees be? _____

7. Banks: Checking Act. No. _____ Safe Deposit: _____
   Savings Acct. No. _____ Credit: _____
   Does anyone else have the Power of Attorney on the above?

8. Final Decisions:
   Do you make them? _____ Or will you consult your wife? _____

XV
CHECKLIST OF
DOCUMENTS REQUIRED FOR ANALYSIS

_____ 1. Business Agreements and/or Employment Agreements
_____ 2. Stock Option and/or Stock Bonus Agreements
_____ 3. Pension and/or Profit-Sharing trust instrument
_____ 4. Deferred Compensation and/or Split-Dollar Agreements
_____ 5. Royalty, Patent, Leasehold Agreement
        6. Owner of Record of:
           _____ A. Bank Accounts
           _____ B. Real Estate
           _____ C. Investments (Stocks, Bonds, Mutual Funds)
_____ 7. Wills and/or Trusts
           _____ A. Revocable Trusts
           _____ B. Irrevocable Trusts
           _____ C. Short-Term Trusts
_____ 8. Social Security Number and/or Government Pension
_____ 9. Insurance policies:
           _____ A. Life — Personal (Self, Wife, Children, Others)
           _____ B. Life — Business, Group, Pension, Profit-Sharing
           _____ C. Accident — Sickness Disability
           _____ D. Professional Overhead Expense Disability

    _____ E. Business Overhead Expense Disability
    _____ F. Hospitalization and/or Major Medical
    _____ G. Liability:

             _____ 1. Personal
             _____ 2. Professional
             _____ 3. Office
             _____ 4. Automobile
             _____ 5. Excess

_____ 10. Amount of last premium and period paid for all policies
_____ 11. Amount of last Dividend and Dividend Option for all policies
_____ 12. Most recent Federal and State Tax Returns

LIABILITIES:

_____ 1. Taxes — Income and/or Real Estate
_____ 2. Amount of Loans — Mortgages, Notes or other Debts
_____ 3. Litigation
_____ 4. Leases
_____ 5.

INDEX

A

Aggression, 133-134, 146
Allopurinal, 94
Amitryptyline, 44
Analgesics, narcotic, 92
Anemia, 126
Anger, 134, 208-210
Anorexia, 126
Antibiotics, 93, 112
Antidepressants, 43-44, 205
Anuria, 76, 120
Anus, imperforate, 156
Anxiety, 6, 8, 38, 107, 118, 127, 129, 134, 143, 153-154, 171, 181, 208, 210-211, 215

B

Bacteriemia, 114
Benemortasia, 75-79
Bereaved
  emotional care of the, 201-206
  medical care of the, 205-206
  support systems for the, 219 (*see also* Grief)
Bladder
  blood clots in, 93
  cancer of, 65-71, 100-102, 110, 111
  contracted, 101
  control of, 90-96
  electric stimulation of, 93
  exstrophy of, 156, 159-160, 174
  infections of, 93
  irradiation of, 97, 100
  neurogenic, 93
  neuropathic, 93
  obstruction of, 115
  replacements of, 93, 115
  surgery, 100, 104, 115
  transitional cell carcinoma of the urinary, 25, 50

Body image, 22, 115, 137, 142-144, 154, 160, 183
Brain dysfunction, 126
Brompton's mixture, 51-52

C

Calculi, renal, 91, 94
Carcinoma, metastatic oat cell, 72
Cardiovascular disease, 113
Catheters, 93-94
  Foley, 72, 94
  Gibbons, 82
Cervix, carcinoma of, 50
Chemotherapeutic modalities, 114
Clergymen, role of, 20-24
Codeine, 51
Colon, malignancies of, 81, 110
Colostomy, 22
Communication, 12, 16, 36, 133, 172, 184, 190
Community hospital, 58-62
Constipation, 95
"Cord" bladder, 7
Cordotomy, 93, 192
Creatinine, 118
Cunningham clamp, 86
Cushingoid facies, 180
Cystectomy, 7, 101, 106, 111
Cystitis, chronic, 101
Cystoprostatectomy, 111
Cystoscopy, 73, 81, 97

D

Death
  acceptance of, 13, 16, 17
  cultural reactions to, 213-214
Dehydration, 91
Dementia, renal, 126
Dementia dialytica, 126-127

233

Denial, 38, 42, 118-119, 134, 140, 155, 163, 172, 181, 196, 207-208, 212
Dependency, 54-55, 125, 136-137, 146, 211
Depression, 6, 17, 38, 45, 51, 107, 113, 117, 119, 127, 129, 132, 134-136, 144, 171, 179, 181, 196, 205, 208
Dextroamphetamine, 57
Diabetes, 104-108
Dialysis, 80-81, 91, 109, 117, 119, 160
  adjustment to, 128-132
  dementia and, 126
  encephalopathy and, 126
  organic brain dysfunction and, 126
  psychiatric complications of, 133-147
  psychological aspects of, 123-147
  psychosocial problems of, 179-185
  stages of adjustment to, 127-128
Displacement, 39, 127, 155, 181, 209
Dysparthria, 126
Dysphasia, 126
Dysuria, 50

E

Edema, 6
Enterostomal therapist, role of the, 25-34, 86
Epispadias, 156
Estrogen therapy, 99-100
Ethics
  biomedical, 80-82
  committees on, 58-62
Exstrophy, cloacal, 177 (*see also* Bladder)

F

Fears, 65-71, 118, 153-155, 164, 172
Fibrosis, pelvic, 101
Financial concerns, checklist, 223-232
Fistulae, 7, 101
Foley catheter, 72-73, 94
Funeral
  primitive society rituals and the, 209-210
  role of the, 220

G

Gastrointestinal problems, 93
Genitourinary tract, carcinoma of, 6
Gibbons catheter, 82
Grief, 17, 119, 130, 201-206
  ambivalence and, 218
  anniversary reactions and, 206-221
  anticipatory, 9, 17, 18, 117-122, 157, 193, 202
  conversion reactions and, 216
  guilt and, 203
  hypochondriasis and, 205, 207
  pathological, 205, 207-221
  physical illness and, 215
  psychiatric complications and, 215-216
  psychosomatic manifestations of, 202-203
Group process, the, 49-57
Guilt, 210-212, 214
Gynecodynia, 99
Gynecomastia, 99

H

Hematuria, 77, 93, 101
Hepatitis, 126
Hormonal therapy, 114
Hospice program, 62
Hypnosis, 192
Hypnotics, 43, 205
Hysterectomy, 115

I

Identification, 39, 205, 214, 216-217
Ileostomy, 22, 26
Imipramine, 44
Immunosuppressants, 118, 160, 180
Impotence, 22, 98, 104-108, 126, 143
  organic, 107, 111
  psychogenic, 107
Incontinence
  fecal, 86
  urinary, 6, 8, 86-89, 94, 95, 164, 178
Insomnia, 209
Intellectualization, 43

K

Ketoacidosis, 105
Kidney
  carcinoma of, 102
  failure of, 126, 128, 159, 179-185
  psychological stages during transplantation rejection, 118-121, 139
  transplant, rejection of, 117-122
Kübler-Ross, stages of dying, 11

L

Levorphanol, 52, 56
Living-dying interval, 5
Loneliness, 9, 217
Lymphatic channels, obstruction of, 6

M

Meningomyelocele, 175
Metastasis, epidural, 99
Morphine, 57

N

Narcotics, 57
  addiction to, 92
Nephrectomy, 7, 143
Nephritis, glomerular, 91
Nephroblastoma, see Wilm's tumor
Nephropathy, diabetic, 91
Nephrosclerosis, 91
Nephrostomy, 75, 78, 81
Nocturia, 99
Noradrenalin, 105
Norepinephrine, 105-106
Nurses, 49-57

O

Oral care, 32
Orchiectomy, 100
Ostomy, 22, 88, 100
Ostomy nursing, 25-34

P

Pain, 56-57, 92, 101, 110, 114, 171-172, 192
Palliative procedures, 115
Pancreas
  biopsy of, 114
  cancer of, 113-114
Paraplegia, 99
Patient
  chronically ill, 123-147
  emotional needs of, 8-12, 174-177
  fears of, 65-71, 100, 144-145, 153-155, 161-162, 172
  geriatric, 113-116
  need to be informed, 189-195
  participation in decision making, 189-195
  pediatric, 153-157, 158-168, 170-173, 174-178, 179-185
  psychological complications, 123-147
  psychological effects of chronic hemodialysis on, 123-147
  psychological evaluation of, 120-121
  psychological status of, 38-40, 65-71, 120-121
  psychosocial problems and management of, 37, 41-44, 47, 113, 179-185
  rights of, 189-190
  terminal, 16, 49-57, 72-74, 78-79, 113-116, 128, 157, 170-175, 218-221
  treatment, right to refuse, 17-78
Pearman prosthesis, 109
Pediatric urology, see Patient, pediatric
Penectomy, 105
Perineal resection, abdominal, 81
Pharmacotherapy, 43-44
Physician-patient relationship, 6, 12-13, 40, 43, 116, 191
Priapism, 109
Primary physician, 35-48, 72
Projection, 38, 155, 181, 213
Prostate, 72, 98-100
  adenocarcinoma of, 25
  biopsy of, 114
  carcinoma of, 92, 98, 100, 110, 112, 113-116
  hormonal management of cancer of the, 99
  metastatic cancer of, 98-99, 101
  radiation treatment of, 97-98
  surgery, 22, 73, 98, 104
  transurethral resection of, 95
  tumors of, 98, 113
Prostatectomy, 7
Prosthesis, penile, 7, 88, 104, 105-107, 109-112
"Prune-Belly" syndrome, 174
Psychiatrists, 35, 49-57
  role of, 131-132
Psychologists, 172
Pyelograms, intravenous, 95, 99
Pyelonephritis, 91

Q

Quinlan committee, 95-60

R

Radiation therapy, 97-98, 114

Reaction formation, 39
Rectum, surgery of, 104
Regression, 10, 39, 42, 133, 136, 155, 179
Rehabilitation, 28, 136
Renal dementia, 126
Repression, 39, 155
Rhabdomyosarcoma, 170

S

Self-esteem, *see* Body image, Self-image
Self-image, 22, 124-125, 133-134, 179, 181, 183-184
Sexual function, 104-108, 109-112
  activity, 26
  fears related to, 68-69, 143, 178
  interstitial implantation techniques and, 98
  loss or diminution of, 6, 7, 110, 136, 143-144
  mechanical restoration of, 109-112
  self-assessment questionnaire of, 106-107
Small-Carrion prosthesis, 109-111
Social workers, role of, 158-168
Spina bifida, 159, 175
Suicide, 117, 137-141, 189, 208, 215
Support systems
  family, 17, 145-147, 153, 157, 166, 182-183
  hospital, 83-85, 160, 165-167
  patient, 43, 100, 153, 156-157, 182-184
Suprapubic tube, 72-73

T

Terminally ill
  estate planning for the, 196-199, 223-232
  (*see also* Patient, terminal)
Testosterone, 105
Tranquilizers, 43
Transsexual surgery, 104
Transurethral resection, 72, 95

U

Urachus, patent, 174
Uremia, 77, 80-81, 126
Uremic encephalopathy, 126
Ureteostomy, cutaneous, 75, 78
Ureters obstruction of, 99
Urethritis, 72
Urinary diversion, 25, 75-79, 80-82, 87
  obstruction, 75-79, 80-81, 99
  retention, 114
Urination, cessation of, 143
Urogenital malignancy
  psychosocial aspects of, 97-103
  radiotherapeutic management of, 97-103
Urologic illness
  cancer, 170-173
  pediatric, emotional effects of chronic, 153-157
  psychological needs and, 174-178

W

Wilm's tumor, 156, 159, 170

DATE DUE